Think
yourself
YOUNG

Think
yourself
YOUNG

Gloria Thomas

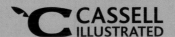
CASSELL
ILLUSTRATED

First published in Great Britain in 2003 by
Cassell Illustrated, a division of
Octopus Publishing Group Limited
2-4 Heron Quays, London E14 4JP

A CIP catalogue record for this book is
available from the British Library.

ISBN 1 84403 013 X

Design and illustrations by
Tanya Devonshire-Jones
Photography by Bill Norton

Printed in Italy

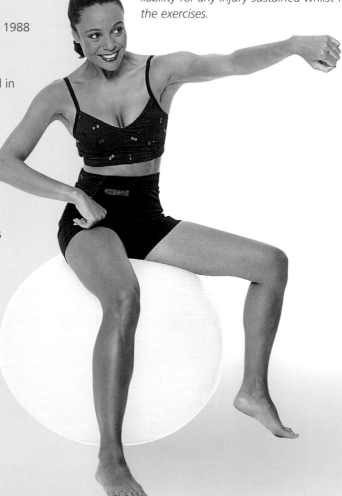

DEDICATION
I would like to dedicate this book to Greg Smit
and Cedric Douse.

Disclaimer – *It is advisable to consult a physician
in all matters relating to health and in particular to
check with your doctor before embarking on any
exercise regime. While the advice and information
in this book is believed to be accurate and true at
the time of going to press, neither the authors nor
the publisher can accept any legal responsibility or
liability for any injury sustained whilst following
the exercises.*

Contents

Introduction

'I dread getting older', 'you can't teach an old dog new tricks', 'your body grows old against your will', 'leopards don't change their spots'. Are any of these statements true for you? They used to be true for me. I used to believe that growing old would be a painful process with stagnation setting in once you got past a certain age. Like everyone else, I have been brought up to categorize people at different stages of life. I used to believe that growing old should be avoided at all costs. But I now believe that this thinking is the result of a collective mindset that is backed up by mediums such as film, television, radio and magazines that purport that it is better to be younger.

However, my actual experience about ageing tells me something very different. As I constantly work towards my own personal development in mind, body and spirit, I have found that the biggest things I have learned is how beliefs have such a profound effect on our lives. They set the boundaries and guidelines that we live within regardless of whether they empower and dis-empower us. It is our collective beliefs about ageing that have actually created a society with a fear of growing old and prejudices such as ageism.

Yet other cultures have a more empowering view of getting older. In some societies it is believed that as you get older, you get better. With this belief, as people age they are encouraged to do more to be active and independent in mind and body. They integrate well with the younger members of society. Wisdom and experience is revered.

It is time now to challenge our existing beliefs on ageing. This book is completely relevant to young and old. I now believe that it is how you live your life that is most likely to determine how you age. We have so much influence on how we can do this. You can literally create more youthful cells in your body by addressing the way you think, which changes what you do. It is psychological and biological age that counts. Time now to throw away your everyday calendar and think yourself young.

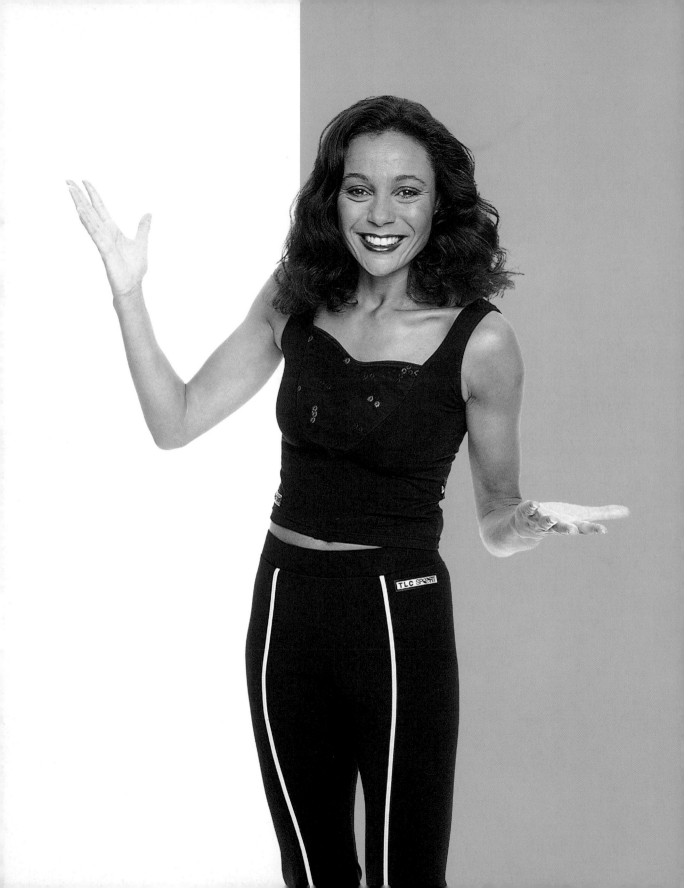

Chapter 1

Exploring Age

What does being younger mean to you? Does it mean looking younger? Being more beautiful? Having more energy and vitality? Being able to sprint at top speed for a bus? Feeling great about yourself? Getting your guitar or drum kit out of the cupboard again? Or does it mean avoiding getting older with the general decline and degeneration that occur over time?

Exploring Age

We are a nation with a fear of getting old. This fear comes from living in an ageist society that believes ageing is something to avoid rather than celebrate. Film, television, magazines and newspapers inform us directly or indirectly that it is better to be young. And there are big bucks to be made out of this fear. Carefully planned advertising campaigns scream at us to buy products to bury the wrinkles on our faces or cover the lines on our necks that date us like rings on a tree. The shelves are full of products that will put back together the bits of us that are falling apart.

At all levels of society assumptions are made and people are put into categories according to their age – in the work place, at home, in the spheres of sport and leisure. Science and technology advance at great speed and are seen as exclusively for the young. Western society assumes that there is less to look forward to as we become older and that retirement means you should relax, put your feet up and do less. It also assumes that getting older means a general degeneration of both the mind and body.

It is in fact stagnation that causes ill health not old age. If we don't use our faculties we will lose them. It is not using our minds and bodies and the attitude to ageing prevalent in our society that leaves us little hope for our future as we age. On top of this we have become a transient society, with family members living farther and farther apart. Being old can mean being isolated and alone. Is it any wonder that one in five of the older population are diagnosed as suffering from depression?

Yet we have created and contributed to this fear ourselves through what can only be described as 'collective conditioning'. What we think today about ageing is the product of the beliefs of past generations. In the same way, these inherited beliefs affect our ideas about the way we should look, the way that we should act and the way that we should live our lives. When we accept those beliefs we reinforce and impose them on ourselves: 'I'm 35, which is far too old to take up football.' 'I'm 40, which is too old to wear a mini skirt.' I'm 60, which is too old to start playing golf.' 'I'm 80, I should be in an old people's home.'

**If you don't use
your faculties you
will lose them.**

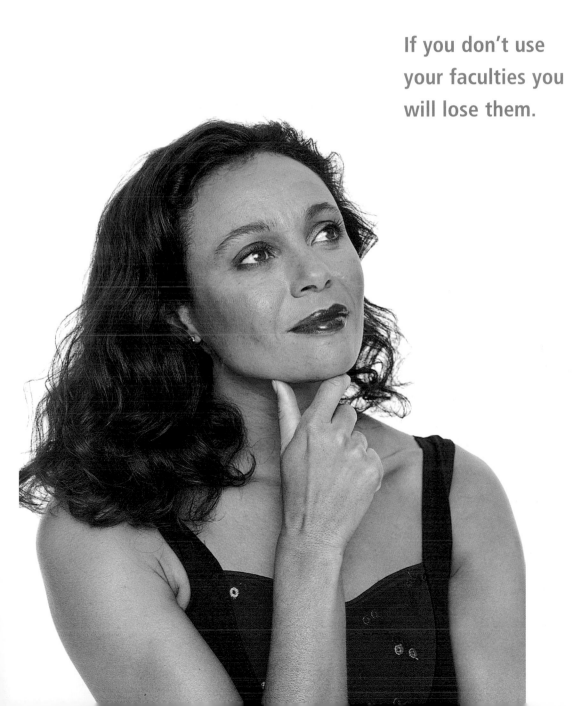

How do we condition ourselves in this way? Human nature is such that we need to make sense of our world in order to function on a day-to-day basis and we need guiding principles by which to run our lives.

We take in information through our senses, which we analyse and store in our minds along with our memories. What we perceive to be true creates our reality and forms the basis of the mental maps that guide us. So what we take in over a period of time becomes our reality. We accept and respond to the messages we hear around us. What we feel we become. Our bodies are the end-product of this process.

Mental Maps

What you currently think about ageing is a result of your conditioning and forms your metal map. Your map may be a positive one, offering a solid route with clear destinations. However, you may have a map that has weak routes and a destination that is confused and unclear.

What is so amazing about the human species is that we have an incredible capacity for change. If you are not happy with your map you can recreate it by simply changing the way that you perceive and think. Alfred Korzybski, in his book *Science and Sanity*, coined the popular phrase 'the map is not the territory', meaning that we all have the capacity to see the world differently and that you can make a new map if you choose to.

Other societies shape their worlds very differently. For example, the people of Abkhasia, a mountain region in southern Russia, expect life to get better and better as they get older – people look forward to old age. A study of centenarians on Okinawa, Japan, revealed that 'age exaggeration' is rampant. The reason being that with old age comes prestige. Qualities such as wisdom and experience are invaluable and place older people higher in the hierarchy. There is a great feeling of being valued, which breeds a sense of purpose and optimism.

In many of these societies you see a different physical expression of age, with centenarians walking and climbing and swimming and performing martial arts. This is in part because the people in these societies have lacked the mod cons of the West, such as easily available transport. The consequences of a greater reliance on the body are an upright posture, strong bones and muscles and considerably fewer of the diseases that have been related to lifestyle in the Western world. Add to this the fact that the extended family is more likely to live together – young and old interact to create a more youthful atmosphere.

Challenging Ageism

Ageism in Western society needs to be challenged as much as sexism and racism. If you choose to continue to accept society's attitudes to ageing you will be made to feel old. You will find yourself behaving older than you actually are. You may ask, how can I change the thinking of others? Well, the truth is you may not be able to do so directly, but you can change yours, which will have an affect on you and those around you. It will take time to change the collective conditioning that afflicts a society and creates its preconceived notions about ageing. You can start by taking responsibility for yourself.

So how do we define an individual's age and how does our current collective view of ageing relate to science? To begin with, your age can take three 'forms'.

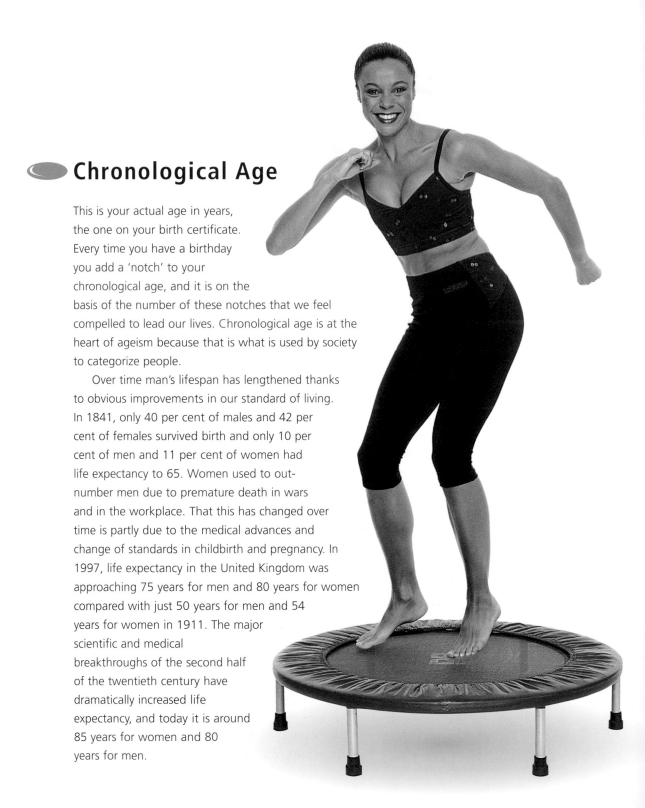

Chronological Age

This is your actual age in years, the one on your birth certificate. Every time you have a birthday you add a 'notch' to your chronological age, and it is on the basis of the number of these notches that we feel compelled to lead our lives. Chronological age is at the heart of ageism because that is what is used by society to categorize people.

Over time man's lifespan has lengthened thanks to obvious improvements in our standard of living. In 1841, only 40 per cent of males and 42 per cent of females survived birth and only 10 per cent of men and 11 per cent of women had life expectancy to 65. Women used to out-number men due to premature death in wars and in the workplace. That this has changed over time is partly due to the medical advances and change of standards in childbirth and pregnancy. In 1997, life expectancy in the United Kingdom was approaching 75 years for men and 80 years for women compared with just 50 years for men and 54 years for women in 1911. The major scientific and medical breakthroughs of the second half of the twentieth century have dramatically increased life expectancy, and today it is around 85 years for women and 80 years for men.

*Write
a list of different areas in your life
where you use your chronological age. Has
it been helpful or harmful? Has your
chronological age prevented you from
achieving any of your goals in the
past?*

Centenarians

According to demographers the number of people who live until 100 is increasing all the time. There are 20,000 people over the age of 100 in the USA today (those who live to 110 are 'super-centenarians'). Okinawa, Japan, is famous for its centenarians. While there are 10 centenarians per 100,000 people in the USA, in Okinawa there are 34. The greatest recorded age reached by a human – a French woman, Jean Calment – was 122 years and 164 days. She died on 4 August 1997 having outlived 17 presidents and taken up fencing at the age of 85. The oldest age a man has lived to is 120 years and 237 days – Shigechiyo Tzumi from Japan. He is said to have worked until the age of 105. Two of the most famous centenarians were the Japanese Kin ('Gold') and Gin ('Silver'). When they each reached their 100th birthday in 1992 they called a press conference to remind people to respect the elderly. At the age of 105 they were still celebrities, giving interviews and making numerous television appearances.

 # Biological Age

Your biological age is the age of your physiology and of your internal organs. It is a measurement of how well your body is functioning. This may conflict with your chronological age, which proves the inaccuracy of the latter as a means of defining age. Your biological age is influenced by genetics and your lifestyle. In youth, your biological age and chronological age may be the same, but as you grow older and your lifestyle and expectations change they can diverge. If you live a particularly stressful life, are inactive and have a poor diet, you are likely to look, and your internal organs may be, older than your years. If you have balance in your life and are physically active and eat nutritionally sound food, the cells in your body are likely to be younger than your actual years. A glamorous grandmother aged 50 could have younger internal organs and look younger than an unhealthy, undernourished and overweight 30-year-old.

For many years disease was asscociated with age. However, there is much research to suggest that in fact disease has little to do with old age and far more to do with lifestyle. Many health problems, such as heart disease, strokes, high blood pressure, diabetes and osteoporosis are avoidable, as are mental conditions such as senility, depression and Alzheimer's. You can maintain your mental and physical faculties if you use them well and even decrease your biological age by 12 to 15 years.

Fertility

One consequence of greater life expectancy is that women are fertile longer. Women can now wait before having children, and many are choosing to do exactly that. Rosanna Dalla Corta of Viterbo from Italy, gave birth, with the help of fertility treatment, aged 63. Studies show that many centenarian women have given birth after turning 35. This suggests that these women's reproductive systems aged slowly, and that on the whole they aged biologically slowly too.

So, your biological age shows how well your body is functioning. And what you need to remember is that poor posture, lack of activity, poor nutrition, stress and the way you manage your life affect the physiology of your body.

Your Cells

All living organisms are made up of cells. Some consist of only one cell but your body consists of hundreds of millions of cells – one quadrillion at a rough estimate: 1,000,000,000,000,000 – all too small to be seen with the naked eye. The cells in your body are combined together like paving stones. Cells mass together to create tissue and form the organs in your body. Inside you are at least twenty different types of cell each with a different job. Smooth muscle cells bring about movement, nerve cells conduct messages from the brain and white blood cells defend the body

Get your kit off and look in the mirror. What is your biological age on the outside? Does your biological age and actual age match up? Think of people you know of the same age and compare their biological age to their actual age. How do they differ?

against disease. The cells in your body are constantly changing and reproducing throughout the whole of your life, even when you become older. The rate of production is greatest in the skin, blood, intestinal wall and your bones. On average your skin replaces itself once a month; the same time it takes your blood to renew itself; a new stomach lining is produced every five days and a new skeleton every three months. It is deep inside the mechanism of these cells that health and vitality begin or fail.

Biological Inheritance

Your biological inheritance – the influence of your parents and forebears – is passed on to you via the chromosomes in DNA (deoxyribonucleic acid). DNA contains a set of coded instructions telling an organism how to develop. In fact, your DNA holds the 'instructions' for the colour of your eyes, how long your legs will be, whether you will be naturally fat or skinny, the colour of your hair and skin. Within each cell there is a genetically coded blueprint for the entire organism.

Leonard Hayflick, a researcher from Philadelphia, developed what is called the Hayflick Limit. His theory states that cells are preset to last a certain length of time. He came to this conclusion by experimenting with human embryonic cells. He could not get these cells to multiply past a certain limit: as they approached their fiftieth division the cells divided more slowly and finally died. Hayflick endorsed the idea that ageing is controlled by a biological clock: as cells approach the end of their allotted lifespan they become susceptible to disease. (Of course, if human cells were to keep reproducing, we would never age.)

Over a lifetime our cells become damaged and they do not always repair themselves. They then cease to function efficiently. The factors that influence this process can be put down to genes or lifestyle factors such as environment and stress.

Although time has an effect on all your cells there is much you can to slow the body's biological processes. Awareness is the key.

Psychological Age

Perhaps the one factor that has the most marked effect on how you age is your psychological outlook on life. While Hayflick explored ageing at a cellular level in a laboratory, ageing guru Deepak Chopra claimed that the whole is far more important then the part, saying that 'your DNA is influenced by every thought, feeling and action'. His contention is that it is the quality of your life, what you think, the way that you handle stress, that affect how quickly the cells in your body age.

Your psychological age, then, is the age that you feel and is influenced by your state of mind and your attitude towards life. The way you think can have the effect of either accelerating the biological ageing process or slowing it down. If your natural state of mind is pessimistic then this has an effect on your body. Depression and different states of pessimism, such as anxiety, anger and worry, send messages to your organs and can have a damaging effect on your immune system. At a cellular level your organs are more likely to become older and you are more likely to die younger.

How you deal with stressful situations will also affect your body at a cellular level. Deal with them badly and you will find yourself pumping stress hormones such as cortisol into your body. And prolonged stress can do a great deal of harm. But perhaps you are optimistic in life and positive in stressful situations, and you naturally search for happier states of mind and see the fun side of life. In which case you will have a very positive response at a cellular level, flooding your body with 'happy hormones' such as serotonin and endorphins and so on. You are likely to slow the ageing process, living a longer, happier and healthier life. Memories also trigger positive or negative feelings, resulting in happy hormones or stressful ones. So you can understand why people only want to remember the good times!

The relationships you have with yourself and others also affects your biological age. If you are self-absorbed or if you talk harshly to yourself, you will find yourself constantly stressed. If you are hard on others, overly cynical and inflexible, you will end up alienating yourself. Harshness, criticism, cynicism and inflexibility result in tension and stress for you as well as others. A healthy relationship with yourself is the basis for healthy relationships with others and vice versa, and both have an effect on how well you live and age.

So your body is very much affected by what is going on in your mind. In fact Chopra goes a step further. In his book *Ageless Body, Timeless Mind* he says that the mind is actually in the body and not in the brain alone. 'Every cell in the body is a non-local mind' and every cell can make 'brain chemicals'. The chemicals that he is referring to are neurotransmitters. These, the body's chemical messengers, determine moods and temperament and have been shown to be responsible for excitability in dreams and hallucinations and for pain regulation. Neurotransmitters distribute information throughout an organism – whenever a thought arises these chemicals 'deliver' it to all the cells in the body. Neurotransmitters are believed to underpin all brain function and it is now thought that they bridge the gap between mind and body.

Here are two lists of some of the factors that can affect how you age. Of these, which tell you most about your psychological age? Any factors from Group A need to be resolved, while any factors from Group B need to be reinforced.

Group A

Depression

Anxiety

Loneliness

Poor communication

Anger

Self-criticism

General pessimism

Lack of fulfilment

Financial uncertainty

Lack of physical affection

Inflexible behaviour

Limiting beliefs

Self-absorbtion

Group B

Optimism

Humour

Great sex

Good communication

Fulfilment at work

Intuition

Flexible behaviour

Calmness

Happiness

Financial security

Empowering beliefs

Affection

Selflessness

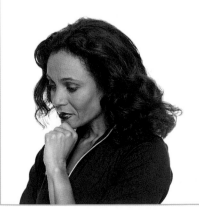

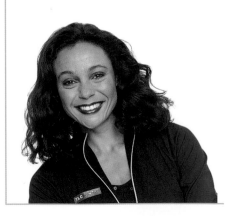

Case Studies

George

George came to me with a chronological age of 55. He had a girlfriend whose chronological age was 35. They got on fabulously well on a mental and emotional level. There was a lot of laughter and a deep level of understanding between them. When he was with her he felt as young as her. However, George had become aware of the physical differences in age, which caused him to worry about the long-term prospects of the relationship. And he did not know where to begin to help himself bridge the apparent age difference. There were a number of lifestyle factors that he had to consider. He was a smoker and he seemed to get out of breath quickly. This would imply that his heart and lungs were older than his actual years. He didn't drink alcohol and drank a lot of water, which would have probably given him younger kidneys. But he was completely inactive and the result was that his muscles had atrophied. He also held a large amount of weight around his waist, the classic middle-age spread. His skin looked like it had suffered from too much sun but, all in all, he looked his chronological age. George's real problem was his lack of belief in his physical ability to do something about the age gap. He wanted to make changes but believed that he was too old. However, the desire to be with his girlfriend helped him to be open to change.

While George had a young mentality he had neglected his body with the predictable consequences. This neglect was the result primarily of a lack of confidence. So, when George visited me, his chronological age was 55 and his psychological age was 35, but his biological age matched the former.

I convinced George that there was a lot that he could do to help himself, and he seemed keen and determined. I suggested a healthy eating plan and regular exercise four times a week. Nine months later George was well on the way to retrieving his muscle mass and had lost his

The best anti-ageing tool is your mind.

paunch. He moved with greater energy and vitality and had given up smoking. Weight training had made his skin tighter and fuller. He looked ten years younger – George had managed to lower his biological age to 45. He had completely changed his thinking about his capabilities and had decided to take up long-distance cycling and mountain climbing. He was successfully working towards his girlfriend's chronological age.

Anna

Anna is 30-year-old housewife who lives in Hounslow. She has three young children under the age of seven. She smokes 20 cigarettes a day and considers her life very stressful. Her relationship with her husband is strained. They don't communicate well and she says that she is lonely. She comfort-eats convenience foods and is around three stones overweight. Anna is woken up by her children a couple of times a night on average. She never plays with them because she is too tired. She also complains of pains in her joints. Anna believes that she doesn't have to address her lifestyle yet – she's too young. But in fact she looks considerably older than her years.

Clearly Anna is allowing herself to age prematurely. Her lifestyle is a result of her inability to communicate with herself and others around her. Already her biological age is surpassing her actual age, which is a result of her being limited and inflexible in her thinking and this is apparent in her unwillingness to address her lifestyle. If she wants to look and feel younger, the first step may be for her to learn how to communicate better with her husband; and she needs to find ways to have a little break from her children. Although her actual age is just 30, Anna looks 40 but her inflexible attitude puts her at about 50.

I remember my 40th birthday and a number of friends offering sympathy and commiserations – and yet I felt great. I was so much wiser and balanced than in my 20s and 30s. I also remember my aunt ringing up to speak to my mother only to find that she was out walking. I proudly told her that my mother would go out walking for up to two hours. 'Ooh no,' she said. 'Be careful, she's 66.' Yet biologically my mother looked and felt better than she had for years when she was taking those walks. One of my best memories of growing up is of my favourite next door neighbour working in the garden in her 80s – laughing, chatting, behaving like a woman half her age. She was clearly a lady biologically and psychologically younger then her years.

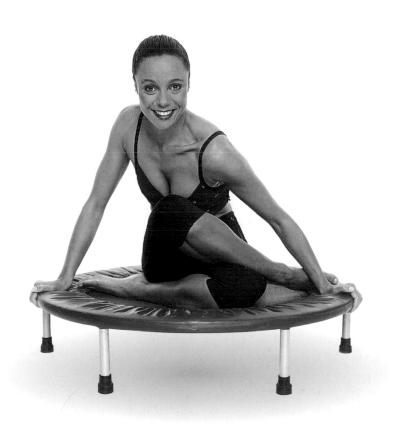

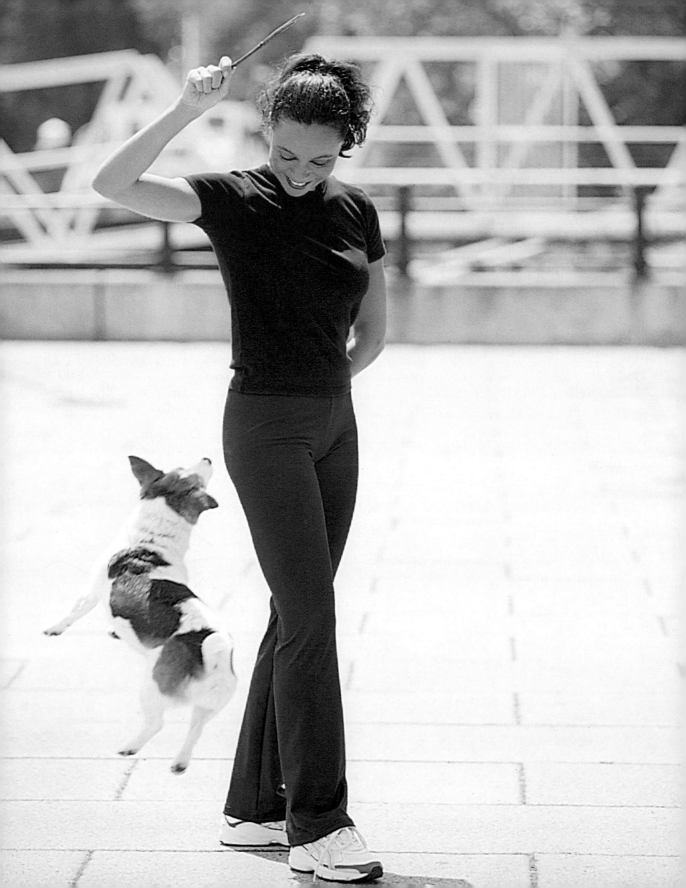

How Well Are You Ageing?

The following simple questionaire explores the last 10 years of your life. Add up your points and see how you do.

Biological Age

How well do you look today compared to 10 years ago?

(3) I look better than I did 10 years ago.

(2) I look the same or a little older than I did 10 years ago.

(1) I look much older than I did 10 years ago.

How is your physical fitness compared to 10 years ago?

(3) I exerise consistently 3–5 times a week and my fitness is the same, if not better.

(2) I exercise some of the time and I am beginning to lose my fitness.

(1) I am now completely inactive.

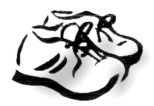

How is your nutrition and eating habits compared to 10 years ago?

(3) I still only eat fresh foods that are good for my body.

(2) I eat more convenience food than I used to.

(1) I only have time to eat convenience food.

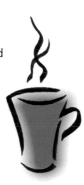

How is your body fat compared to 10 years ago?

(3) I still have the same levels of body fat as I did 10 years ago.

(2) My body fat has slowly increased over the years.

(1) I have put on a lot body fat

How are your energy levels compared to 10 years ago?

(3) I have just as much energy and vitality as I did 10 years ago.

(2) I have less energy than I had
   10 years ago.
(1) I have very little energy.

Psychological Age

How happy do you feel
   compared to 10 years
   ago?
(3) I am very happy with my life
   compared to 10 years ago.
(2) I simply get on with life.
(1) I was much happier 10
   years ago. I don't have
   much to look forward to.

What do you believe about
   getting older?
(3) I believe that as time goes
   by my life gets better and
   better.
(2) I believe that the ageing
   process is inevitable.
(1) I really worry about getting
   older.

How are your mental
   faculties compared to 10
   years ago?
(3) I do a lot to stimulate my
   mind and my concentration
   and memory are better

than 10 years ago.
(2) I read the paper and
   sometimes see the news.
(1) I do very little to stimulate
   my mind.

How do you cope with stress
   compared to 10 years
   ago?
(3) I seem to handle situations
   in a much more calm and
   relaxed way.
(2) I still handle situations in
   the same way that I
   used to.
(1) I seem to get more
   stressed than I used to.

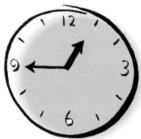

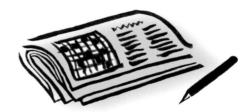

How do you think you have performed in this questionnaire? Add up your points in each section and evaluate each one. Have you improved more in one section than in the other? Are the both about the same. Clearly the more points you have the healthier and happier you are becoming with time. The less points you have, the more useful it may be for you to think about the areas of your life that you need to work on for a more youthful mind and body.

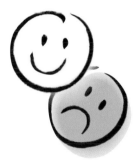

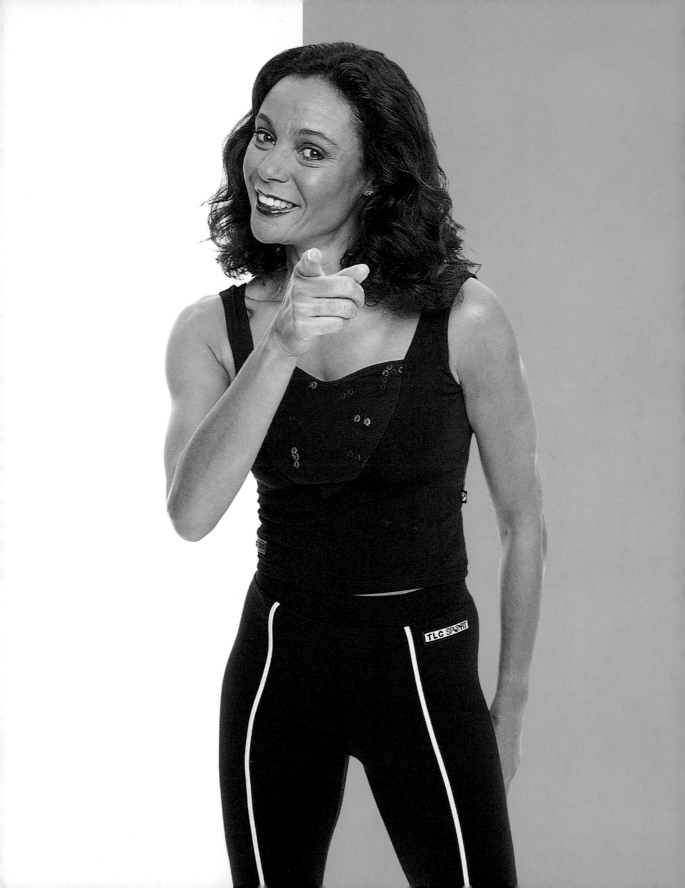

Chapter 2

Your Self-image

You are reading this book because in some area of your life you want to feel younger – mentally, physically or perhaps spiritually. But before imposing super-youth on yourself with the mental and physical exercises that follow, a little self-exploration into the you that wishes to become younger may be helpful.

The person you are today, both mentally and physically, is the sum total of your thinking of yesterday and the person that you wish to be in the future. If you are not happy with way you are ageing it may be useful to explore your experience and see what has made you the way you are today so that you can make changes for tomorrow. Begin by asking yourself these questions: who is the you who wishes to be younger? Will becoming younger fit in with who you really are?

Your Self-image

Your Mental Blueprint

In the same way that DNA holds the blueprint of your physical manifestation, you also have a mental blueprint of the person that you are and wish to be. This blueprint is made up of your likes, dislikes, beliefs and values. This blueprint is your self-image and it has a great influence over the decisions that you make in every area of your life. Your self-image is the product of all your experiences in life. I was born in Ashford in Middlesex, I went to St Michael's Primary School, I loved reading Enid Blyton books, I loved writing stories, I had a red bicycle, I hated rhubarb. Ideas, behaviours and possibilities that don't fit in with your self-image will not make their way into your life. Your self-image develops into a framework to create a picture of yourself as you understand and believe yourself to be.

Mental Chatter

You may not be aware of it but you talk to yourself all the time. It is this mental chatter taking place just beyond your conscious awareness that heavily influences your self-image. Your self-talk constantly gives you feedback as you experience life, labelling events, analyzing and creating opinions of what you like and dislike, and setting personal limits.

Sit in a comfortable position in which you can completely relax. Close your eyes. Imagine that you are in a room with a magic mirror on the wall. See yourself facing this mirror and looking into it – be aware of the image that is reflected back at you. As you examine the image watch as it changes into a younger you at different ages and in different situations. Look at each age or situation as it comes up. Don't make any judgements, just observe. Do this for around five minutes. And then slowly take a deep breath and open your eyes.

Now write down your thoughts about the self-images that you saw in the mirror.

Where does this self-talk come from? In *What to Say When You Talk to Yourself* Shad Helmstetter wrote that 'during the first 18 years of your life you were probably told "no" or "can't" 148,000 times by parents, teachers or through social conditioning'. Although completely unintentional it is this negative programming that forms most of our self-talk. So it stands to reason that the more positive your conditioning the more positive your self-talk is likely to be. But self-talk can be incredibly harsh, critical and self-deprecating and often quite irrational.

And how do you know when you are talking to yourself? Well sometimes you hear just a word or a very short statement. These thoughts feel like automatic reflexes and at first seem very difficult to stop. Self-talk often contains words or phrases like 'should' or 'have to'. Here are a few examples of negative self-talk relating to age.

- 'Grow up and act your age.'
- 'I shouldn't be doing this at my age.'
- 'I look ancient.'
- 'You're not young enough to do that.'

Over the next few days be aware of any self-talk relating to your age. Then take ten minutes to jot down what you've heard. What sort of things do you say to yourself? What do you think about ageing generally and how do you relate those thoughts to yourself?

How did you get on? (Congratulations if you have a positive attitude to ageing.) Did you find that the self-talk was almost automatic in nature? Self-talk is usually reactive and reflects past experience. Although it seems like it is impossible to stop the self-talk, over time the exercises in this book will make you more adept at intervening and preventing negative age-related inner dialogue.

How Does Your Mental Chatter Affect You?

One of the prime functions of the subconscious mind is to work towards the goals that you give it be they positive or negative. It automatically provides the motion or the force to make something happen, so when you talk to yourself you are in fact guiding and directing your mind to establish a reality based on that inner dialogue. If you keep on making comments such as 'I'm not fit enough to …' or 'I'm too old for that' or 'My memory is so poor' you are actually suggesting that your mind should make those very things true. In his book *Sports Mind*, top sports psychologist Jeffery Hodges says, 'You are the person you are today because you keep telling yourself every minute of every day precisely who you are.'

Mental Chatter and Physiology

If your mental blueprint is full of fear and misgivings about ageing, if you limit your decisions about your life on the basis of your chronological age and think 'old' thoughts, then you may find that you age before your time. It is important that you remember that self-talk has its consequences at a cellular level and that your body is a reflection of what is going on in your mind. Doctors and medical researchers say that as many as 75 per cent of patients' illnesses are mind related. If you constantly tell yourself that you are stressed then you'll become stressed. If you tell yourself that you are forgetful you will be. And if you convince yourself that your family's history of heart disease means that you will die at a certain age, you are creating the possibility that this might happen.

Awareness

So how can you learn to change the programming that might have aged you prematurely? You can begin by becoming aware of the dialogue going on inside you. When you are conscious of your self-talk and you awaken to what is being said and why, you open up to the potential for change.

Think of some of the people you know who are rigid in their thinking, who limit themselves to what is known and familiar to them. Think about some of their limiting beliefs – 'I can't do ABC because of XYZ.' But you know they really could do ABC if they were open to change. Now imagine how their lives would be different if they were to let go of their limiting beliefs. Write a list of different areas in your life where you use your chronological age. Have your beliefs about chronological age been helpful or harmful to you? Make a commitment to throw away your everyday calendar and focus on thinking yourself young.

Your Self-image and Beliefs

Your self-image changes over your lifetime in response to new experiences. It is your perception of these experiences, the way you think about your life, the beliefs that you develop, the way you handle life's hurdles that make a difference to the way you age. Much research has been carried out on groups of people who have aged well and they all report that the key to staying young is to believe whole-heartedly that youthfulness is attainable whatever your chronological age.

Before we move on to the tools that will change your self-talk for ever, it is essential to direct your awareness to your existing beliefs about ageing and the beliefs that you would like to have. Because unless you fully understand what these existing beliefs are it will be difficult to change them. Think about the first exercise with chronological and go back to those areas in your life when you use your chronological age.

As time goes by you become the person that you have conditioned yourself to be. You might have conditioned yourself to be a flexible individual open to change and new possibilities. If this is the case, thinking yourself young will come easy to you. But many people have told themselves to be rigid in their thinking, set in their beliefs and determined to stay that way. The result is that they become the living walking, talking, proof of those limiting beliefs.

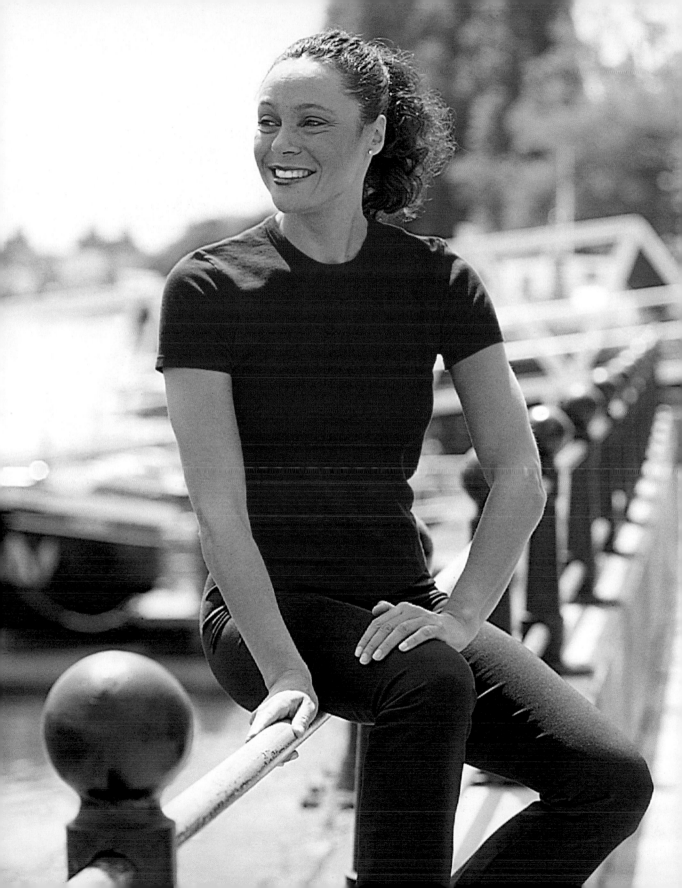

Your Expectations

Our beliefs are wrapped up in our expectations, which influences our behaviour in such a way as to make what we expect to happen more likely to happen. If your beliefs are positive and empowering then that's all well and good. However, if your beliefs limit you it may be that you fear disappointment and therefore expect little, which makes you feel secure and comfortable. Your behaviour and the choices you make can become limited to match those beliefs. Or it may be that the beliefs you have developed are completely false but because you expect them to happen they do. This is called a self-fulfilling prophecy. And it is the same with your expectation of ageing. If your preconceived notion is that we age against our will, or if you falsely believe that ageing means you can expect to degenerate, you will. You'll be thinking yourself into old age.

Case Study

John wanted to become a public speaker. He reasoned that he could easily get up on stage and give a lecture on his chosen subject. After all, he was an expert. However, he also believed that he just couldn't do it because he knew he would mess it up in some way. He was completely convinced that he would sabotage his performance.

The result was that his fearful belief stopped him from even attempting to achieve his dream.

The body will not do what the mind does not believe.

Changing existing negative beliefs is not always easy and you can experience resistance along the way. For example, you may still have old beliefs about age even though they may no longer be relevant to you. Wanting to become younger may not fit in with your existing self-image. Although you look and feel more youthful than you are, you may be using your age as a deterrant. For example you may feel that because you are 40 having a relationship with a

Explore your existing beliefs about ageing. Do they limit or empower you? Are they positive or negative? What do you expect to happen as you go through the process of thinking yourself young? How can you be even more open to the belief that you can make changes in your life? All human behaviour is purposeful even if that behaviour is negative. If you still feel resistance you need to explore why. Limited thinking has its own purpose, perhaps allowing you to fit in with the other people and thus enjoy a sense of belonging or satisfying a need for boundaries and control.

If you do have any existing beliefs that are limiting you write them down now. Ask yourself, 'What is the purpose behind this belief?' You may limit yourself by believing, for example, that 'I am far too old to learn to think myself young.' The issue behind that belief could be that you just don't believe you are capable of thinking yourself young. And the issue behind that belief could be that you don't even have the confidence to begin to try. So, ultimately, the purpose of your belief is that it allows you stay comfortably where you are and not risk failure by trying something new.

30 year old is out of the question as they are far too young for you. You may say that you want to become younger but lack the time or inclination to put yourself through the process. You may question whether it is at all possible to achieve a younger you. You may even be concerned about the new behaviours you'll develop if you are successful. If you are limited in your thinking and create resistance in some way then becoming youthful may be harder for you. However, if you have an open mind, you want to

Ask yourself this question: how can I be even more open to believing that I can become younger?

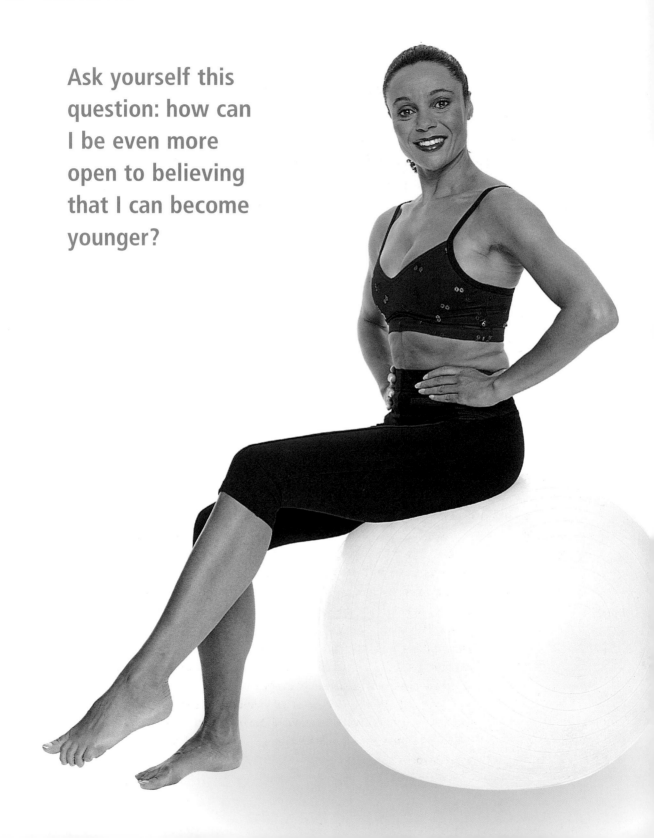

How do you find positive ways to honour the purpose behind an existing belief? For example, if 'staying comfortable' was the purpose behind a limiting belief, ask yourself how you can be confident about doing something new and positive and stay comfortable at the same time? So what you want are ways of looking and feeling younger that won't challenge you too much. How about going to see a funny film that puts a smile on your face. You could listen to some motivating music that will make you feel lighter and more lifted. And you can start to address your weight and fitness levels in a very gentle way – perhaps you could begin with a 15-minute walk every day.

look and feel younger and you make the time to apply yourself to the processes involved, then you will bring about a positive change.

It is important to honour the purpose that generates resistance but, rather than remaining stuck where you are, you need to and can transform it into something more positive.

As you explore new possibilities you will find a level that suits you. Changes can be made at a pace that fits in with who you are. As your expectations change you will find that your behaviour will begin to become more flexible. This will give you a great sense of freedom and youthfulness and you can mould yourself into the person that you want to be, sidestepping any resistance that comes your way.

If you really want to think yourself young it is essential to expect and believe that you will be successful. Now that you have opened your mind a little more it may be useful to understand how your beliefs are formed.

What is a Belief?

Your thoughts are impulses of energy shaping and forming all the time in your mind. It is the acceptance of these thoughts that forms opinions and suggestions into firm beliefs. Beliefs are unconscious patterns that determine how you structure your experience. In other words how we filter and format our experience of the world around us. Your beliefs become generalizations that underlie your thinking and you automatically establish a reality out of what you believe to be true. Beliefs can also be completely without logic.

Consider the following story by American psychologist Abraham Maslow. Believing that he was a corpse, a man went to see a psychiatrist. The psychiatrist tried in vain to reassure him that he was very much alive. But the man was adamant. The psychiatrist asked, 'Do corpses bleed?' The man replied, 'Of course corpses don't bleed.' The psychiatrist told the man that he would prove to him that he was alive and, with the patient's permission, pricked his finger. 'I see,' said the man. 'Corpses do bleed.' The message behind this is that beliefs can be completely illogical and very hard to shift when someone is convinced by them. If you are determined to believe something, no one can change your thinking except you.

Core beliefs are generally formed in childhood from the suggestions and ideas that are fed to us from the world around us – our parents, teachers and peers. You can imagine how beliefs in different nations can form conflicts. Imagine a history lesson on the same event taking place in two different countries that have opposing views about something. Imagine the scene with the teacher explaining to the children 'the facts'. Do you suppose that both teachers are giving the children the same information? The information given can form and shape the beliefs of the child.

Beliefs are incredibly powerful and what you believe can make a difference to your success in life. It is belief that can make the difference between perfect health and poor health and it is belief that will activate the resources that allow you to become a younger you.

Beliefs and Biology

Your body reflects your thinking and every cell in your body responds to your beliefs. The stronger the belief the more ingrained in the body it can become. This has huge implications for health and the ageing process.

A classic example of how your beliefs affect the body is shown by the placebo effect. The placebo is an inert substance that possesses no 'real' medicinal properties yet has the power to cure because the patient believes in its healing abilities. It has been estimated that over 50 per cent of patients respond positively to what is essentially a belief pill! The expectation that one is going to get better activates the individual's internal resources and this is responsible for the improvement. A placebo is any 'treatment' that mobilizes individual expectations. In the First World War wounded soldiers were told that they were to receive a powerful new drug that was even more effective than morphine. They were injected with water and responded to it as if it were the super-morphine. The effect of a placebo is to release endorphins into the body; these are the body's natural painkillers which lead to a sense of well-being.

Emile Coué, pharmacist and creator of the affirmation 'Every day in every way I am getting better and better', discovered the power of the placebo when a customer visited his shop to complain that his medicines were ineffective. Coué made up a concoction that was essentially a placebo and told the patient that it was a marvellous new drug with amazing healing powers. A few days later the man came back cured of his condition.

There are many other instances of the power of belief. Religious belief in a higher being can completely shape an individual's life by establishing boundaries and guidelines for behaviour. The practice of voodoo in certain societies has resulted in 'unexplained' deaths – it is now thought that the victims of voodoo were so convinced of the power of the ritual that they were literally frightened to death. The ancient Egyptians had sleep temples to which people would come with their ills and troubles. The priests would

Think about and make a list of your own everyday placebos. For example, every glass of water you drink you whole-heartedly believe that this will make you feel more youthful and healthy.

induce a trance and tell them that they would be better when they woke up. The Egyptians believed in the divinity of the priests to such an extent when they awoke they were 'cured'.

Perhaps even today we have not really shaken off our totally unjustified fear of hypnosis. (Stage hypnotists have not done much to quash this fear.) There is a belief that the hypnotist has some kind of power over the individual, or that the state of hypnosis is a supernatural one. This is far from the truth. All hypnosis is self-hypnosis, and nobody can force a person to become hypnotized. Hypnosis is a natural state of mind that you achieve every day of your life just before you go to sleep and just before you fully awaken in the morning.

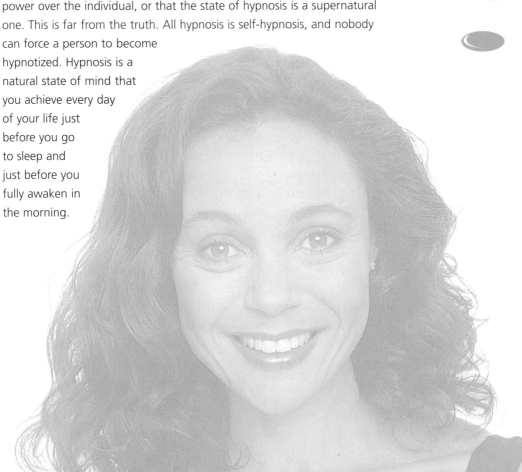

Western society believes that your body and mind grow old and decline and that you have no choice in the matter, that ageing is an unpleasant experience mentally and physically. There is no doubt that changes take place over time that affect mind and body, but it is how you allow yourself to age that results in a biologically and psychologically older or younger you. Often disease and disability and low states of mind are mistaken for old age. All of these can be addressed. The truth is that ageing is very much an individual thing. It is how you believe you will age that not only makes all the difference to the way you look and feel but to your longevity as well.

For many years society has been telling elderly people to put their feet up and rest. But gerontologists at Tufts University carried out a strength study on a group of people over 80 years of age. They were put on a strength-training programme for two months. The results were amazing. Muscles that had severely atrophied over the years came back to life again and after two months frail individuals who were unable to walk unaided could push themselves out of a chair and walk around. Studies such as this have done a huge amount to convince elderly people of the potential of regular exercise.

Changing Your Beliefs

What you believe about ageing will affect your body's biological age for better or worse. But how can you transform your existing negative beliefs about ageing? The previous exercises should have shown you that a mindset open to new beliefs is most likely to begin the process of change. The next step is to further question the validity of your current negative beliefs by finding counter-examples to prove yourself wrong. The more you doubt your old beliefs the more open and receptive you'll be to new ones.

The central props of your belief system, which themselves will have been coloured by your conditioning, are 'reference experiences'. They

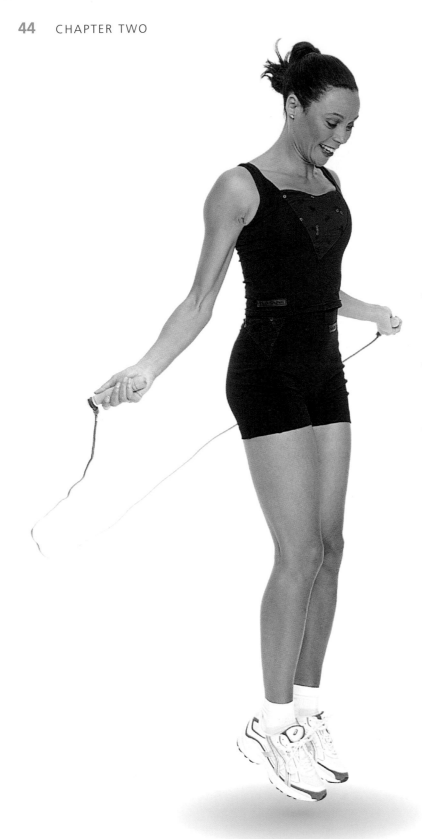

Your body does not age in the way that you have been led to believe.

What are your current reference experiences about age? Write down five reference experiences? Where did they come from? Are they positive or negative? If they are negative, do you still want to hold on to them? Find positive reference experiences to prove yourself wrong and doubt the validity of the old belief.

might have been drawn from your own life experience, and they may be positive or negative. You hold them up to prove to yourself that your beliefs, even your false beliefs, are true. An example of a negative reference experience, therefore, might be, 'I know that I'm not going to enjoy getting older: just look what happened to poor Mrs Smith.'

There are some great positive reference experiences of individuals who have got better as they got older; many are entertainers who are frequently in the spotlight. Madonna, now in her 40s, has a magnificent ability to adapt herself to the times – she looks great and her music is still high in the charts. Jane Fonda, now in her late 50s, has successfully maintained a flexible career that has taken her from acting to politics to fitness guru. Sean Connery, 70 in 2000, is regularly voted one of the most desirable men in the world. Tom Jones, born in 1940, and Mick Jagger, born in 1943, still possess considerable sex appeal. Joan Collins, who will be 70 in 2003, has what can only be described as an indomitably youthful spirit. She claims that her youthfulness and longevity in an ageist business can be put down to the firm belief that age is just a number. (And her present husband is 32 years younger than she is. She believes passionately that there are no age barriers when it comes to love.)

It is interesting to compare Joan with Cher, who of course had a hit with the song 'If I Could Turn Back Time'. Cher, born in 1946, has maintained a youthful image throughout her career, but she has spent a lot of time under the surgeon's knife (and paid a lot of money for the privilege), and her obvious fear of ageing has brought her a great deal of media attention. She says that in her industry becoming old and becoming extinct go together hand in hand, and it is becoming extinct (not necessarily old) that she finds unattractive. That sounds a bit like a limiting belief to me. Yet, and regardless of the cosmetic surgery, she still has a formidable voice matched by few of her younger rivals and an 'attitude' that is undeniably youthful. Tina Turner in her early 60s looks likes a woman 20 years younger then her chronological age. Jerry Hall bared all at the age of 46 in the play The Graduate. The list goes on.

In case you think that these people have simply pampered themselves young, here is a list of people whose achievements are the result of effort and self-belief alone.

- Astronaut John Glenn Jr was a member of the crew of the space shuttle Discovery in 1998 – when he was 77 years old.

- William Ivy Baldwin crossed the South Bolder Canyon in Colorado, USA, on a tightrope on his 82nd birthday.

- Brian Blessed is the oldest man to have climbed Everest, doing so at the age of 64.

- Dimitrio Yordanidis was 98 when he ran a marathon in Athens in 1976.

- The oldest woman to complete a marathon was 82-year-old Thelma Pitt Turner of New Zealand.

- US Golfer Hale Irwin was 45 years and 15 days old when he won the US Open in 1990.

- Margaret Du Pont of the USA won the mixed doubles at Wimbledon when she was 44 years and 125 days old.

- Lynford Christie was a grandfather when he competed in his last Olympics.

- Lester Piggot was 59 when he retired from horseracing.

You no longer need to live up to the expectation that degeneration and decay are inevitable.

And it seems that the beauty industry is beginning to comprehend that all the anti-ageing creams in the world will not turn back time. The beauty market now has its 30-plus role models such as Liz Hurley and Cindy Crawford. Lauren Hutton, born in 1943, Isabella Rossellini, born in 1952, and Carole Bouquet, born in 1957, are all instantly recognizable figures. At 85 Coco Chanel was still the head of the fashion house she founded.

Neither is age a bar to creative expression. At 90 Pablo Picasso was producing drawings and engravings. At 88 Michelangelo devised the architectural plans for the church of Santa Maria degli Angeli in Rome. Vladimir Kandinski, abstract painter and part of the Bauhaus movement, took up painting in his 40s. At 93 George Bernard Shaw wrote the play Farfetched Fables. Winston Churchill wrote his History of the English-Speaking Peoples when he was 82.

Who else can you add to these lists? And what has made these people youthful throughout their lives? The answer is their empowering beliefs. If you have limiting beliefs about age in any context – work, relationships, beauty, sport, leisure – you will find that you will live out those beliefs and make yourself older than your actual years. But all of the people mentioned above have set examples for you to emulate.

What Would You Rather Believe?

You may no longer desire to hold your current beliefs about ageing but what are you going to replace those beliefs with? You can begin by thinking about creating beliefs that are in line with how you want to be. You can take control and create your own empowering beliefs about ageing to match the self-image that you desire. Remember that beliefs are self-fulfilling prophecies and that having a new belief will create change in your behaviour and your physiology.

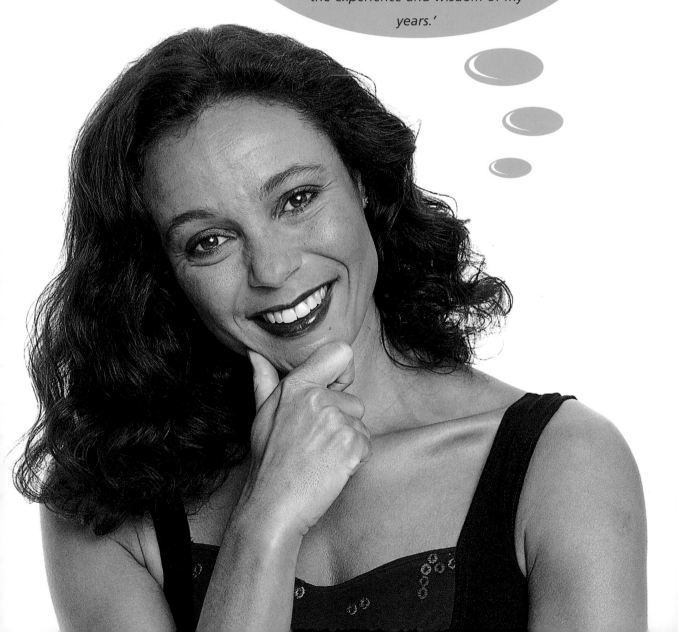

Get some colourful pens and jot down what you would rather believe. For example, 'I can have a biological age of 33', 'I can be more youthful in the way I move', 'I can have loads and loads of fun', 'I can be flexible in my behaviour', 'As I grow older life will get better and better', 'I will retain the experience and wisdom of my years.'

Identify with the age that represents the mental and physical capacities you would like to have and keep. Decide on the age of your younger self. Choose a time 10 to 15 years ago – it should be a time when you were in good health and enjoying life. Get yourself into a comfortable position in which you can completely relax. Imagine that you are looking into a full-length mirror and that you see your younger self reflected in the mirror. Imagine that you get up and walk over to the younger you in the mirror.

Now imagine that you step into the mirror and into your younger self. Open your eyes and move about as the younger you. Become that younger self – see, hear, feel, even smell and taste as he or she would.

This exercise will assess and evaluate your motivation to realize this younger you; it will tell you if you believe it is something worth pursuing. Rate your degree of belief in response to the following statements on a scale of one to five, where one indicates a very strong belief.

- Being younger is desirable.
- It is possible to achieve this younger self.
- It is worth the time and the effort that I am going to put in.
- I have the internal resources to do it.
- I deserve to reach this outcome.
- I can maintain a younger me.

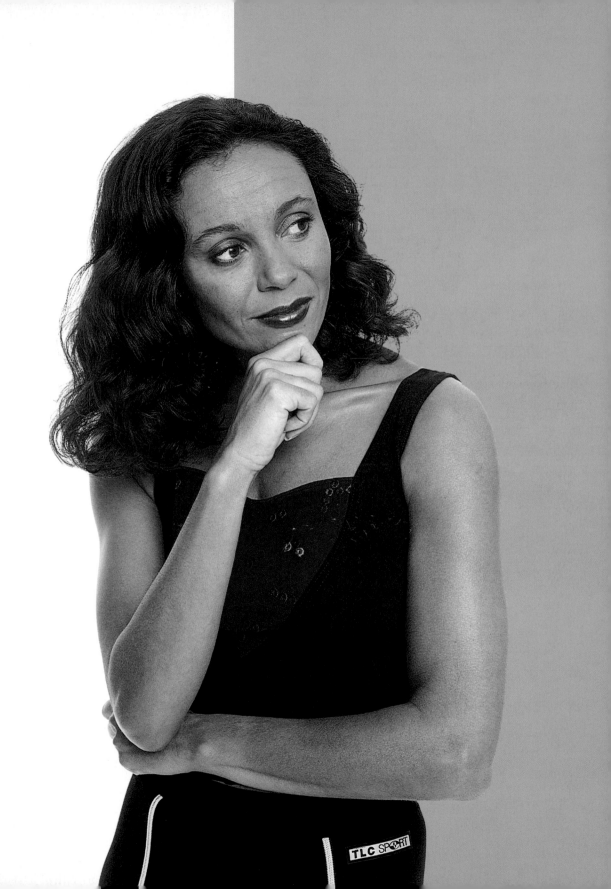

Chapter 3

Learning How to Change

You have had much to think about while exploring your current beliefs about the ageing process. And you now understand that you have become the person that you always believed yourself to be. You have explored your mental blueprint and you know that your self-image is the product of your programming, and that you might have conditioned yourself to age prematurely. But it is time now to focus on the future and to fuel the belief that you would rather have: that with age you can grow younger and better, that youthfulness is attainable whatever your age. It is time now to focus on the tools that will allow you to change your thinking and develop new skills and behaviours and thus achieve your dream of a younger you.

Learning How to Change

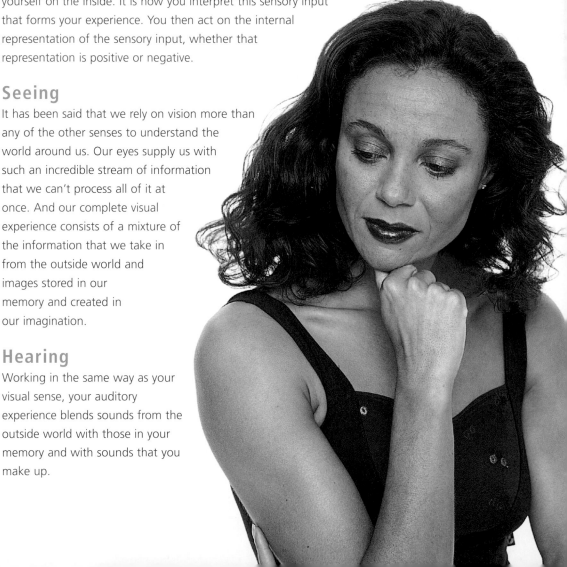

Your Senses

Your thinking affects every cell in your body and is based on the information that you have taken in through your senses. What you see, hear, feel, smell and taste on the outside you then represent to yourself on the inside. It is how you interpret this sensory input that forms your experience. You then act on the internal representation of the sensory input, whether that representation is positive or negative.

Seeing

It has been said that we rely on vision more than any of the other senses to understand the world around us. Our eyes supply us with such an incredible stream of information that we can't process all of it at once. And our complete visual experience consists of a mixture of the information that we take in from the outside world and images stored in our memory and created in our imagination.

Hearing

Working in the same way as your visual sense, your auditory experience blends sounds from the outside world with those in your memory and with sounds that you make up.

Sit in a comfortable position in front of a mirror. Look closely at what you see – an image looking back at you. Find a point to focus on such as your eyes or your forehead. Spend a few minutes paying attention to what you see. The more fully you focus on what you are looking at the more detail you will notice and be able to represent in your mind. What do you see?. 'I see a strong attractive-looking face with an earnest expresssion. As I look more closely I see brown skin a bit like tanned leather. I see a deep frown line in the middle of my forehead and big brown eyes that seem to have a number of different colours in them. I see eyebrows that are black in colour and fine in texture and eyelashes that are also black but thicker than my eyebrows. I see high cheek bones and skin tight over them but a little loose underneath. I see a mouth slightly open with strong white teeth.

Now recall an image of yourself when younger. Spend a few minutes looking at the picture in some detail. For example, 'I see a picture of myself at nine or ten years old. What stands out is the colour of my eyes. I clearly have a big gap between my front teeth. My forehead and skin are smooth. The colour, shape and texture of my eyebrows are black and I have a happy little smile on my face.

IMAGINATION: Now close your eyes and recall the image that you have just seen of yourself in the mirror. Bring all the details that you liked from the picture in the past – smooth forehead, tight skin and a happy smile. Now imagine bringing these qualities to the image of you as you wish to be in the future – youthful, vibrant, warm and happy.

Sit in a comfortable position and close your eyes to enhance your experience. Listen to the sounds that you hear around you. What can you hear? Your internal dialogue? Sounds coming from inside and outside of you? Now speak for a few moments and listen carefully to your voice and tonality. 'I hear a lot of noise around me – the chatter from the people on the balcony next door. I can hear both male and female voices. I am also aware of the washing machine and as I speak I am aware of the depth and gentleness of my voice.

Now close your eyes take yourself back in time to a pleasant experience. What do you hear? For example, 'I am a member of the school choir and we are singing one of my favourite hymns. My voice is strong and deep if a little tremulous, and its pitch sometimes changes without warning. We are singing during school assembly so I can hear the rustle of music sheets and the odd cough and comment from staff and children.'

IMAGINATION: Now imagine you are bringing the qualities of the younger you to your present sound. Notice the difference. I hear my voice change slightly. It has more laughter in it. It has an interesting ring to it. It is less gentle and more playful.

The way we process information on the inside can often be seen on the outside through observing the eyes. These are known as eye accessing cues. The pictures on this page give others a clue as to how we are thinking. These are generalisations and are not true in all cases.

1 Images we make up.

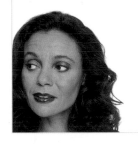

2 Images we remember.

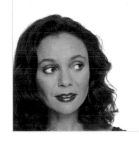

3 Sounds we make up.

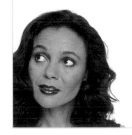

4 Sounds we remember.

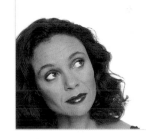

5 Feelings and senstations.

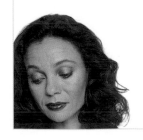

6 Internal dialogue.

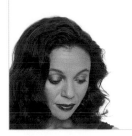

Imagination is more powerful than reason.

Feeling

We all know how powerful the memory and imagination can be when it comes to feeling – what it is like to remember or anticipate (or even fantasize) so vividly that the feelings are real (which of course they are). So just as with your visual and auditory senses, what we feel is a product of the outside and inside worlds.

We have explored what you currently see, hear and feel around you and the sensations of remembered experiences. You have also seen that it is possible to imagine realistic sensations and that your sensory experience is not just visual but auditory and feeling as well.

Your imagination creates your reality. What you imagine yourself to be, you become. If you create positive images and hear positive self-talk your body will work towards these goals. However, if your mind is full of negative images and inner dialogue then you will act to make these real.

Sit in a comfortable position. Your eyes can be either closed or open. Imagine that you have the younger self-image that you desire. See yourself ten years younger then your current age. Hear your voice as if it were ten years younger. Imagine what it feels like to be ten years younger.

How you use your imagination will generate success or failure in your life. You can harness it – you can prepare your inner world to match the outer world that you desire. You do this by imagining the younger you that you wish to be – always focus on what you want and not on what you don't want – and then fine-tuning your senses so that the picture is as complete and detailed as possible. This powerful image can further enhance your motivation to reach your goal.

You get what you focus on.

You may find that you have a preferred sense. There are a number of ways of establishing which is your preferred sense. Did you find one of the 'seeing', 'hearing' and 'feeling' exercises above harder or easier than the others? That may tell you whether you are a visual, auditory or

Still sitting comfortably, take your awareness to your body and the sensations you feel. What does the temperature of your body feel like? Do you feel any tightness or tension in your limbs? Where exactly do you feel this? Do you feel any pressure in your body? What is the intensity of this pressure? How is your breathing? Is it deep or shallow? Do you hold your breath? Can you feel your heartbeat? Jot down what you felt. For example, 'My body feels warm. My muscles are a little tense and my hands are bunched into fists. I feel myself holding my breath a little and then breathing deeply.'

Now take yourself back to a positive experience that you had when younger. Allow the feelings to come back to you and put a label on them. To help you, you may need to remember the sights and sounds of the experience and then step into it. For example, 'I remember the feelings that I used to have on the athletics track. A wonderful feeling of freedom as I ran and ran. I had a sense of lightness and joy and freedom in my body. My body felt powerful and strong. I loved the feeling of the wind against my skin. My breathing was controlled and relaxed.'

IMAGINATION: Imagine yourself as you wish to be: a more youthful you. See a dynamic moving picture of youself using your body in a fit and youthful way – maybe on a brisk walk or jogging. Bring all the feelings of freedom and lightness from this experience to this picture of you. Step into the picture and try on these feelings. Now think of other feelings you would like to capture and add them to the picture. Allow the feelings to get bigger and bigger. As the feelings peak, think of a word or a symbol to associate with these feelings so that every time you use this word or symbol these postive feelings flow into your body.

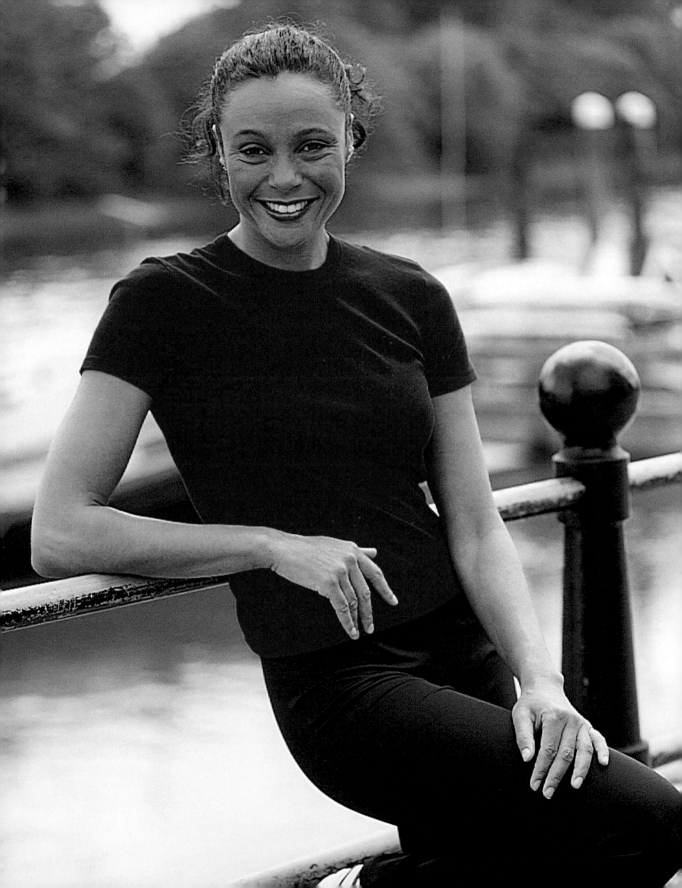

Always focus on what you want.

kinaesthetic (feeling) person. You can also look at what you do for a living and what you do for enjoyment in life. For example, a visual person will probably choose a profession such as graphic design and enjoy the plastic arts. For them the important thing about being youthful may be looking younger. If you are a feeling person you are likely to choose a profession such as nursing or some form of physical therapy and perhaps enjoy massage and physical contact. Becoming younger is most likely to be about feeling younger and developing more youthful behaviour for you. If your dominant sense is auditory then your profession could be one that requires public speaking or you may be involved in music or journalism, and you will probably enjoy listening to the radio. Youthfulness for you may be about sounding younger and using younger language. You can also get an idea of which is your dominant sense by listening to the language you use. Expressions such as 'You look your age', 'A sight for sore eyes', or 'I feel like I'm a hundred', 'He's a real pain in the neck', or 'I sound old and cranky', 'I hear you loud and clear', suggest, respectively, a visual, a kinaesthetic and an auditory person.

Problems may arise if one sense is considerably weaker than the others. For example, you may find it difficult to visualize a younger you toward which you can work. You may find that you are not aware of your internal dialogue or that you are not in touch with your feelings. You can strengthen all your senses if you choose to by simply paying attention to them and using them more consciously.

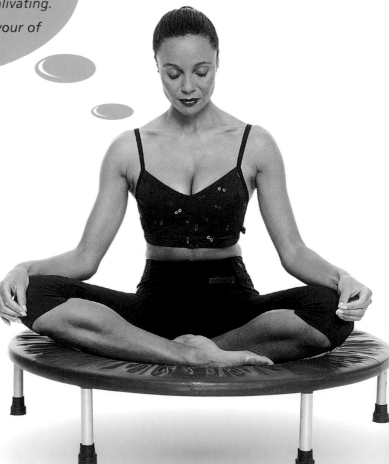

Sit in a comfortable position. Imagine that you are sitting at a table with a lemon, a knife and a plate. See the colour of the lemon, its shape and size. Imagine yourself picking up the lemon and what it feels like – its waxy texture. Smell that citrus aroma. Put the lemon down on the table and cut it in half and then quarters. Watch the juice run from the lemon as the knife cuts through it. Imagine yourself lifting the lemon to your mouth and biting into it. Taste the lemon and savour the flavour of it. Be aware of the sensations in your body as you taste the lemon.

How was that? There are a number of typical responses to this exercise. Some people get a real sense of the tartness of the lemon, others find themselves salivating. Others experience the real flavour of the lemon.

You can make a difference to the way that you get older.

A Physiological Response

Our bodies respond at a cellular level to the images that we create in our minds. Just as it responded to the imaginary lemon as if it were real. So each time you picture yourself getting older or think of yourself getting older or label yourself an old person, your body will respond to this.

Studies have shown that mental imagery can have an affect on the muscles of the body. It has been proven that visualizing a movement activates the same neural pathways as performing that movement for real. And many athletes, businessmen and even politicians use mental imagery to achieve and enhance their goals in life. Athletes, for example, will visualize every moment of a race in minute detail in order to anticipate what they will have to do to win.

Untapped Potential

So what is all of this telling us? Simply that what the mind focuses on tends to happen and that how you use your mind will play a large part in determining the results that you get in life. You have inside of you the most incredible untapped resource and you have the potential to achieve so much more than you think you can.

In the past you might have allowed limiting beliefs and negative thinking to control you. But you now realize that you can cultivate your sensory experience, that you can refine your imagination and guide your mind to create your own desired reality. You can achieve all your dreams in life, and you can take control of the ageing process in all the cells in your body.

Your Experience

How you use your imagination will make a big difference to your experience. The more refined your senses are and the more precisely you use them, the greater the effect on the physiological processes in your body. The senses have been described as the building blocks of your experience. Within the main 'modalities' – seeing, hearing, feeling, smelling and tasting – are still smaller building blocks that make up the quality of experience. These are called sub-modalities and they are responsible for the finer distinctions of your experience. For example, you can encode a visual experience in bright and vivid colours or in dim and dull ones. The more vividly you see hear and feel an experience, the greater the extent to which the body responds.

The following lists comprise a number of sub-modality distinctions. Add to them any more that you can think of.

Visual	Auditory	Kinaesthetic
Associated/dissociated	Volume	Movement
Brightness/dullness	Continuous/discontinuous	Intensity
Black and white/vividness of colours	Tempo	Frequency
Location and distance of objects inside the image	Clarity	Light/heavy
Depth (two- or three-dimensional)	Stereo/mono	Pressure
Still/moving	Sounds	Temperature
Contrast	Tonalities	Location (where in the body or on the skin you feel)
Framed/unbounded	Location (where the sound comes from)	Texture
	Distance (how far away the sound comes from)	Duration

Recall a pleasant experience and, as it comes back to you, be aware of how you represent it. What colours do you see? Notice the location of the image in your mind – is it near or far? Look at the contrast of it. Look at the depth. What do you hear? Are you hearing 'loud' or 'quiet'? What about pitch? Does what you hear seem far away or close by? Where is the location up, down, side or straight ahead.

Now be aware of how you feel as you relive this experience. See if by altering the various sub-modalities – the colours, the distance, the sound and so on – you can change the intensity of your feelings.

As you further explore your experience you will see that you can exert a great deal of control over it. You will find that you can change negative states to positives, that you can enhance your feelings to motivate yourself to work towards a younger you. The optimum state in which to think yourself young is a relaxed one. When your body and mind are relaxed, you can focus and clearly guid and direct your internal resources. The following are some of my favourite exercises for reversing the ageing process. The first will show you how to change a negative state of mind or feeling into a positive one.

A Younger Self-Image

When we set ourselves a goal we are in fact aiming to 'create' something in the future. The more precise and specific we can be about that goal, the more likely we are to achieve it. When you focus on what you want you will find that you are driven to find the ways and means needed to reach that goal.

Think of a negative state related to ageing, perhaps anxiety. Close your eyes and think of the location of this feeling in your body. Explore the intensity of this state. If this state were to have a colour, what would it be? Give the state a voice. What is the tone of that voice – is it harsh and loud or quiet and monotone?

Now take each part of this state and change it so that it is how you want it to be. Begin by reducing the intensity of the feeling and adding some warmth to it. Change the voice. If it is hard and harsh, make it soft and mellow. If is a quiet, droning voice that you can't really hear, turn it off completely, or turn it up so that you can hear clearly what you are saying to yourself. And if it isn't positive then change the tone and content of what you are saying. What about the colour? Are you happy with it? Change it to the opposite of whatever it is now. If it is dark, make it light; if it is dull, make it bright. As you make adjustments just be aware of the state changing. When the state has changed to your satisfaction – when everything about the state is just right for you – think of a symbol. Whenever you want to access this positive state, all you have to do is recall the symbol and you will experience a sense of well-being throughout body and mind.

Sit in a comfortable position and breathe deeply as you count down from ten to one. Exhale after each number. When you feel fully relaxed and your mind is clear, bring back the image of you as you wish to be – perhaps ten years younger or at an age that you can realistically imagine yourself to be. Imagine you are looking into a mirror and that you see your younger self reflected in it.

As you look at this younger you imagine a control panel by the side of the mirror. Use the controls to fine-tune the image you see. Explore the texture of your skin, your muscles, the expression on your face. Make the image as clear as you can: you want to see every detail. Make the colours brighter and lighter. Position the image at the right distance away from you or closer to you. Now adjust the sound. How does your more youthful voice sound? Is it higher or lower? What is its tone? Keep working at the control panel until it is just as you wish it to be. As you look at this image, think about how you want to feel. What attitude do you want? Adjust the controls so that you are happy, vibrant, carefree, youthful. Take one last look at the mirror and ask yourself this question: 'Does this image fit in with my sense of self?'

If the answer is 'No' then you need to adjust the controls until you are completely satisfied. If the answer is 'Yes', open your eyes and move about as the younger you. What does it feel like – are you faster, lighter, energized? Is there anything else you want to add to these sensations?

Sit in a comfortable position and associate into an experience of youthfulness. See what you would see, hear what you would hear, feel what you would feel. Now imagine stepping out of your body and floating around the room until you find a comfortable position from which you can observe yourself. How far away do you need to float before you have a sense of total dissociation from the sensations? Have a good look at the younger you before returning to your body.

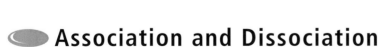

Association and Dissociation

When you associate you are inside an experience seeing, hearing and feeling from your perspective. When you dissociate you are outside an experience looking on. You can still have feelings when you are dissociated but they will be feelings about an event; you don't have a sense of being part of that event. You can use association to experience what your younger self feels like and to monitor those feelings.

Changing Internal Dialogue

'Grow up and act your age.' This is just one example of the harsh self-talk to which we subject ourselves. Now, whenever you hear your inner critic getting ready to sabotage your efforts and your ambitions, make a point of consciously stopping whatever you are doing and addressing it. Listen carefully to the voice and note as many of its characteristics as you can. Now change the voice. Alter its tone, pitch and rhythm. Change the content of what you are saying so that it is positive. Make the voice funny so that you break into laughter whenever you hear it. Model it on the voice of a cartoon character: Betty Boop, Chip and Dale, Mickey and Minnie Mouse – it's entirely up to you. Now choose a fun symbol to represent this new voice – and the next time your inner dialogue becomes negative, think of the symbol and you will immediately be flooded with good-humour.

We mentioned earlier that the inner dialogue we have with ourselves seems to be automatic and it can feel like it is difficult to stop. However, you can learn to intervene. You do this by increasing your awareness and then consciously stopping the negative dialogue in its tracks. You then replace the old dialogue with more positive and useful suggestions.

Sit comfortably and imagine a timeline running from the present to the future. Now take the younger self that you saw in the mirror and place it in a picture frame. See yourself floating above your timeline with this picture in your hands. Place the picture at different points on the timeline – you want to find the time by which you can realistically expect to have achieved that younger you. When you think you've got the right spot, leave the picture there. Now – still on your timeline – fully associate into the picture and ensure that every detail feels right. Step out of the picture and bring all the positive feelings with you. Walk back along the timeline until you get to the present. As you look into the picture of your future, be aware of the sense of well-being that you have brought with you. Feel the connection between you and the picture and use the picture of the younger you as a symbol to bring back all those great feelings at any time in the future.

Sit back and relax. Take a few deep breaths. Start to count backwards from ten to one. Exhale as you count each number and inhale in between. As you count, direct your attention inward and imagine that you are taking a trip inside your body to explore all the cells of which it is made up – your skin, your blood, your muscles, your internal organs, your nervous system. Explore the current condition of those cells and see if there is an area that needs special attention? Have a look at their colour and texture – are they all the same or do they differ? If you were to add sound to those cells, what would you hear? If your cells were sending you a message, what might that message be?

Now think about how you would like those cells to be, how you want them to look, sound and feel. As you do so, visualize beads of life flowing to every part of your body, regenerating each cell so that it is full of vitality. See how the colours of those cells change and come to life. See your nervous system light up like a Christmas tree. Feel youthful energy flowing throughout your body. Hear yourself talking gently to your cells: use warm, encouraging words. You don't even have to talk: simply flood your cells with a healing, youthful sound. Focus now on how you feel as you make these changes in your body. Allow the feeling to be come more and more intense and to get bigger and bigger. As your feelings peak, give yourself a symbol. And whenever you see this symbol in the future your body will flood with rejuvenating chemicals to make all the cells in your body more youthful.

What the mind believes the body will do.

Cell Rejuvenation

You can use your imagination to communicate with all the cells in your body. You now know that every part of your body is responding to your thinking and that your cells are renewing themselves all the time. You know that if you are thinking negatively, you are likely to flood your body with stress hormones. But you can also think positively so that your feel-good chemicals will kick in.

Affirmations

Self-talk is learned. You might have learned to talk negatively about ageing, which has resulted in limiting beliefs and behaviour. However, you can unlearn this and start to use positive language to develop mental flexibility, which will lead to behavioural flexibility. You do this by simply changing the words and phrases you use from negative to positive and repeating them until they become true. Positive statements that are used in this way are called affirmations and they are an extremely powerful means of changing behaviour. Here are some affirmations that you can use in the exercise on the opposite page.

- 'I feel youthful and vital.'
- 'My skin feels younger every day.'
- 'I am calm, confident, relaxed and at ease.'
- 'My muscles are lean and strong.'
- 'I move with grace and elegance.'
- 'My vision of things both near and far is clear and sharp.'
- 'I look 35 years old.'
- 'I am more active as every day goes by.'
- 'My bones are strong and healthy.'
- 'My voice is full of joy and laughter.'
- 'I enjoy eating healthy foods that nourish the cells in my body.'
- 'My energy increases every day.'

Choose one affirmation at a time to work on. Say it out loud and with feeling – like you really mean it. Now create a mental picture of the action that you want to take or the end-result that the affirmation will bring you. Adjust the sub-modalities to create a really compelling image, one that you feel irresistibly drawn towards. Fully associate into the picture and the feelings. Reaffirm the affirmation.

Studies have shown that successful ageing is a result of keeping mental and physical faculties young. One of today's assumptions is that as we get older we become set in our ways and confine ourselves to what is familiar and comfortable. But beware: this can happen at any age. As you work through the exercises in this book you will find that your behaviour becomes more youthful. And as your self-image develops into a more youthful one you will find new behaviours come easily. In the past, you might have believed that as you become older you should do less. But you now know that the less you do the more you age. So, are you set in behaviour patterns that are ageing you?

Laughter has a profound physiological affect on the body; it is even prescribed as part of the cure for many illnesses in Indian medicine. So when you find yourself stuck in a behaviour pattern that makes you feel older you can begin to change the pattern by making your state more youthful. Laughter is the perfect tool with which to achieve this.

Think about a behaviour pattern that has aged you? Recall an experience where you carried out this behaviour. As you relive the experience look at the sub-modalities around this behaviour. Write your response to your experience.

What kind of behaviour do you associate with youthfulness? Use words and images to respond to this question. Look at the sub-modalities in the pictures you are creating and the language you are using.

Compare the sub-modalities of your ageing and youthful behaviour. Now sit back and imagine applying the sub-modalities of the positive behaviour that you associate with youthfulness to any negative behaviours to which you are prone.

Recall an experience that really made you laugh. As you recall the experience fully relive it by associating into the situation. See what you saw, hear what you heard, feel what you felt. Allow the feeling to get bigger and bigger in your body until you want to explode with mirth. Create a visual symbol (one that adds to the laughter) to represent this feeling and just recall it – and with it the feeling – whenever you need an instant lift.

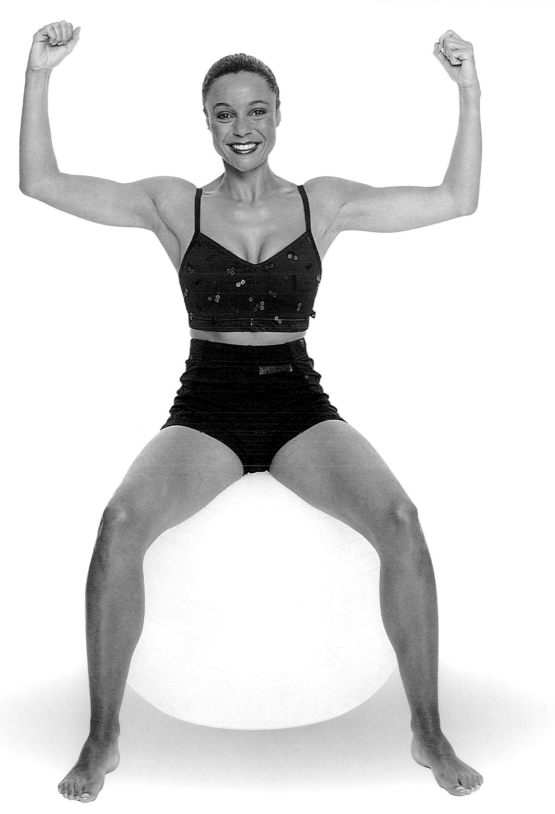

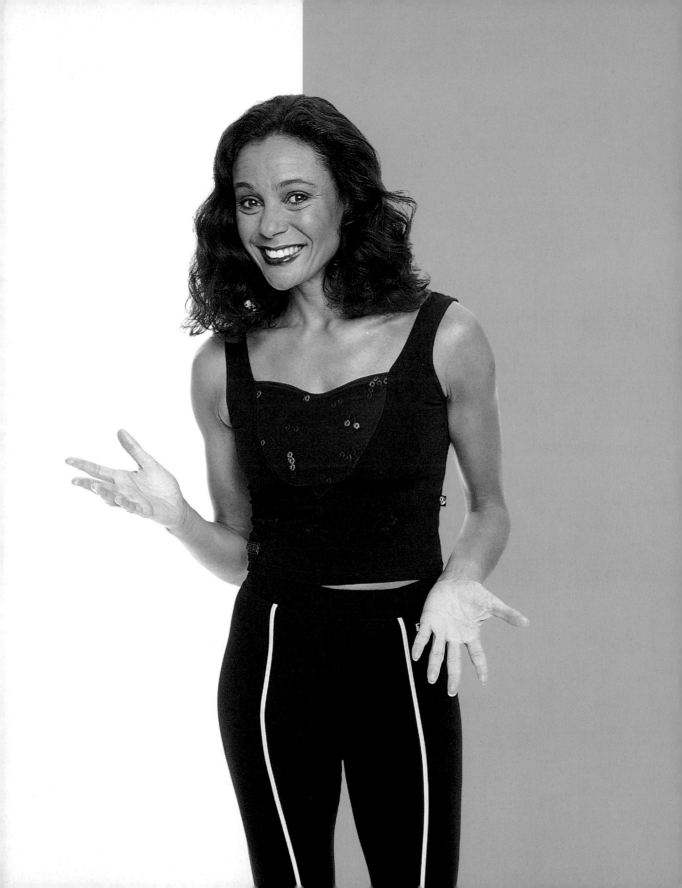

Chapter 4

Your Body and Youth

Human beings are designed for activity. One of the functions of the brain is to control and coordinate movement. In the distant past our ancestors' movements were adapted to the harsh conditions of their lives. They had strong, fit bodies, the result of dynamic movements such as running, jumping, hunting and carrying. Do you think you would have seen an obese hunter–gatherer? I doubt it (at least not one who would have survived for long). And in the past, body fat was there for sound biological reasons: to provide insulation from the cold and energy in times of famine. Today we do not need to insulate ourselves from the cold, nor do most of us have to worry about famine. But we continue to store all that excess energy in our bodies as fat.

Your Body and Youth

In the past, our lives were based far more on physical labour and activity. The land was worked on by hand and machinery that had to be operated manually and people travelled on foot. The technological advances of the twentieth century have – for better or worse – promoted a sedentary lifestyle.

But your body is still fundamentally that of your ancestors, no less predisposed to the movement that keeps it strong and healthy. So, if you don't use your body you will find that it simply won't function as it should; it will degenerate prematurely in a way that we conventionally associate with ageing. But while your chronological age is undoubtedly linked to physiological changes over time, it is your biological age – the one that you can choose to influence – that we are interested in here. Let us start by looking at the effects of time and inactivity on the body.

Your Heart

Your heart is a muscle and like any neglected muscle it can lose its functional ability over time. The cardiovascular system can decline as much as 5 to 15 per cent per decade between the ages of 25 and 70. Your heart rate, measured in beats per minute (bpm), drops every decade by six to ten bpm. (Your maximum heart rate is calculated as 220 minus your age; if you are 25 your maximum heart rate will be 195; if you are 40 it will be 180; if you are 60 it will be 160.) The stroke volume, which is the amount of blood pumped from the heart each time it beats, lowers as you age, as does cardiac output, which is the amount of blood pumped by the heart each minute. Your resting heart rate of 60 to 80 bpm generally stays the same until the age of 60, but your recovery rate slows down. However, activity will quicken your recovery rate and strengthen your cardiovascular system.

To test your aerobic fitness start by measuring your resting heart rate. Then run or walk up and down the stairs for a few minutes. Time how long it takes for your heart rate to return to normal. (Do this one month into a programme of physical activity and see how much more quickly you recover.)

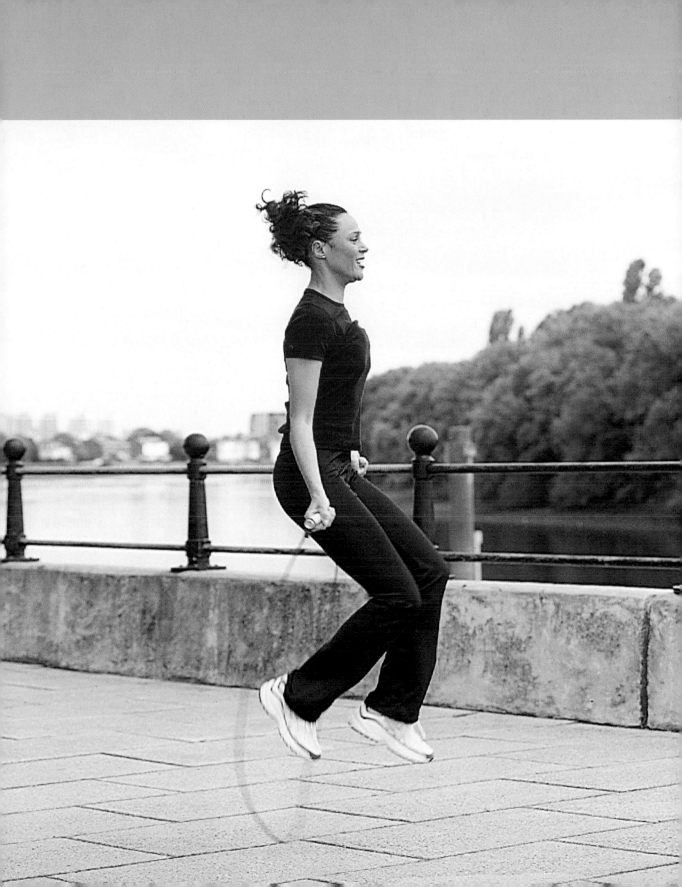

What is the current condition of your heart? Do you exercise it regularly? Do you find that you get out of breath quickly? Can you climb the stairs with ease? Make a decision to develop your awareness of how you are currently using your heart.

Make a list of five ways to increase your VO2 Max. Perhaps, for example, you can walk to the shops instead of driving or throw yourself into your gardening. You could really put your back into the vacuuming or take the stairs instead of the lift.

Your VO2 Max

The aerobic system is so-called because it uses oxygen to produce energy. (You also have anaerobic metabolism that produces energy without oxygen.) Your aerobic capacity or VO2 Max is a measure of your ability (in relation to your body weight) to consume oxygen at a cellular level. A high VO2 Max indicates the increased ability of the heart to pump oxygen-absorbing blood to the lungs and of the muscles to take up that oxygen. Inactivity can mean that your VO2 Max progressively declines by 40 to 50 per cent between the ages of 20 and 60. Physical activity considerably slows this process by much as 5 to 15 per cent over the same period.

Lie in a comfortable position and place the palm of one hand on your navel and the other on your upper chest by your neck. Exhale and draw the abdomen in so that the hand on your navel sinks – but make sure that your other hand stays perfectly still. Hold your breath for a moment before inhaling and allowing your abdomen and ribs to swell. Hold your breath a moment before exhaling.

Now imagine stepping out of your body and watching yourself breathe. Are you breathing easily and naturally from the diaphragm, or are you tense and breathing from the top part of your chest? Stand up and imagine that you are a breathing instructor and allow yourself to coach yourself into position. Do five minutes of breathing every morning and evening.

Your lungs

If you don't exercise your lungs your respiratory efficiency declines. Your breathing muscles weaken and air is not circulated as effectively around your lungs. Sedentary living means that you simply don't fill your lungs with air, something you do all the time if you are physically active. But there are exercises that will work your breathing muscles and maximize the efficiency of your lungs.

Your Muscles

You know the saying 'Use it or lose it', well nowhere is this more the case than with your muscles – they will atrophy if you don't make the most of them. It is well documented that between the ages of 20 and 90 you can lose as much as 50 per cent of your muscle mass. And after the age of 30 there is a decrease in muscle fibre and an increase in body fat. (These changes are most pronounced in women.)

We are all born with two different types of muscle fibre: fast twitch and slow twitch. Fast-twitch fibres are characterized by their quick response to stimulation and are used in explosive movement. Athletes who run in the sprint events have a high proportion of fast-twitch fibres. Slow-twitch fibres have a slower contraction speed and are associated with endurance sports such as marathon running. So if you are, or were, a sporty individual you will probably have a predominance of fast-twitch fibres. In most people the split is around 50:50.

Inactivity and time lead to a reduction in the number of fast-twitch fibres, resulting in a loss of speed and strength in your muscles. For men this means that muscles are less likely to hypertrophy (that is to say, get bigger) in the same way they might have done at an earlier age. And studies show that 40 per cent of the female population in America aged 55 to 64, 45 per cent of women aged 65 to 74, and 65 per cent of women aged 75 to 84 are unable to lift a 4.5kg weight as a result of inactivity. This process can be delayed considerably with strength training.

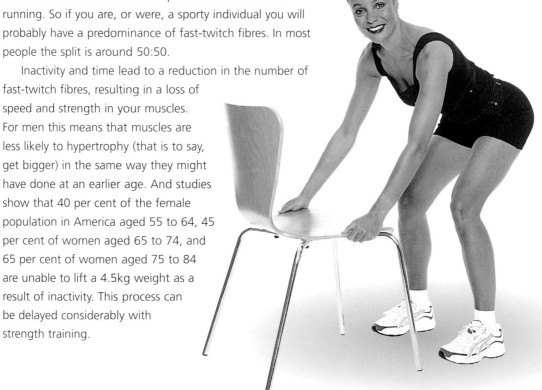

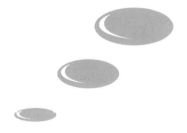

Think about the muscles in your body. Do you use them? Recall a time when your muscles were at their peak – what did they look and feel like? What are your muscles like now? Are you as active as you were in the past? Now think about the future. How much stronger could your muscles be if you were to consistently exercise them? Imagine now what they will look and feel like.

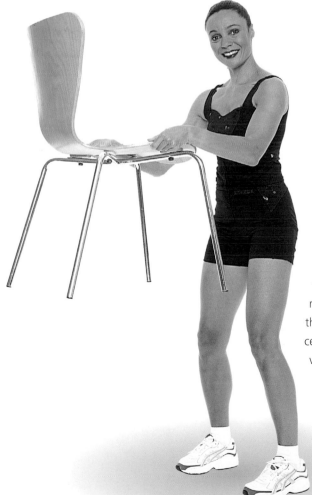

A 1989 study by Tufts and Harvard universities tested sedentary individuals aged between 80 and 90 to determine the heaviest weights they could lift. They were then started on a strength-training programme that involved working out with a weight that was 80 per cent of their respective maximums. At the end of six weeks they had increased their strength by 180 per cent, and many were able to get around without their walking sticks and push themselves out of their chairs without using the chair arms. When the participants returned to their sedentary lifestyles they lost this ability. We can see indisputable proof that you can increase your strength considerably at any age.

Sit comfortably, breathe deeply and count down from ten to one. Imagine a dial that represents your metabolism. Give the dial a colour and number it from 1 to 20. Take three deep breaths and allow a number to come up on your dial that represents your current metabolic rate. If you are not happy with it imagine yourself adjusting the dial to the metabolic rate you want.

Make a conscious decision to imagine your new metabolic rate every morning and evening in conjunction with finding ways to raise your metabolism.

Metabolism

About 60 to 70 per cent is used to maintain your heart beat, breathing and body temperature and to control your body. Your metabolism peaks around the age of 20 and then declines by two per cent every decade thereafter. There are a number of factors that affect it.

Your body composition – what you are made up of: bones, muscles, organs and fat – affects your metabolic rate. Muscle is more metabolically active than fat, so the more muscle you have the more calories you burn. This means that men tend to have faster metabolisms than women. Your body type will also affect your metabolism. If your body type is muscular or very skinny, you are more likely to have a faster metabolism than someone who is prone to putting weight on quickly and perhaps has been chubby since childhood.

As a child the proportion of your body fat is small: 10 to 15 per cent of total body mass. As changes take place in the body during adolescence this proportion can increase to 15 to 20 per cent for men and 20 to 25 per cent for women. Muscle mass begins to decline with time and inactivity around the age of 30, and your metabolism begins to slow down. As your metabolism slows, body fat increases, so that by the time you reach your middle years the proportion of body fat may rise to 20 to 25 per cent for

Your metabolism slows with time and inactivity.

men and 25 to 30 per cent for women. (After menopause a woman's body fat may make up as much as 35 per cent of her body mass.) But just because your metabolism declines, it does not mean that the energy you take in does. So if the energy you take in does not match this declining need for calories you put on weight.

The more of your muscle mass that you can preserve, the more you can help to prevent the decrease in your metabolic rate and combat the ageing process. You preserve muscles mass through strength training. You can also guide your imagination to find ways to increase your metabolic rate.

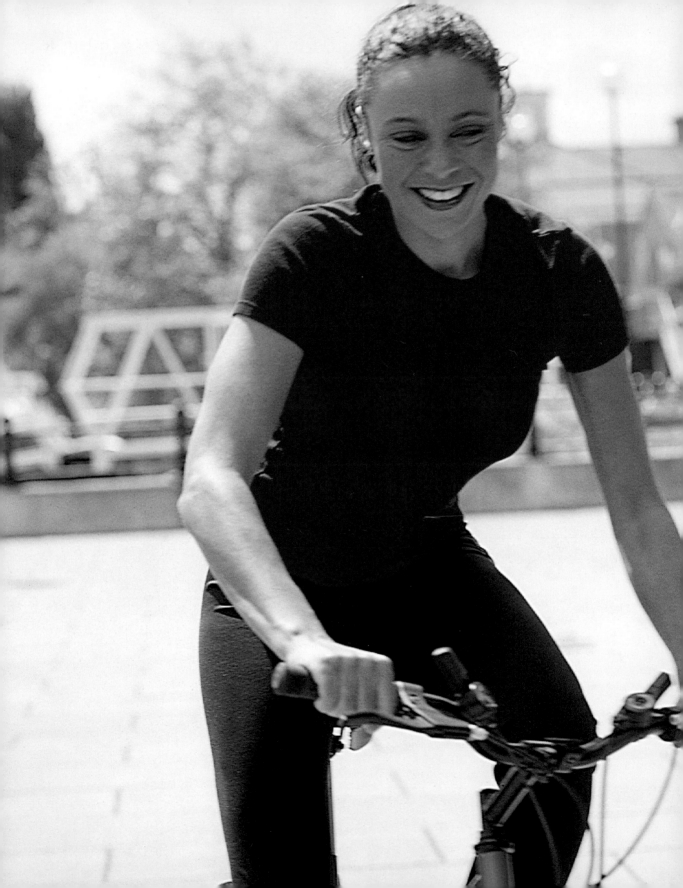

*What
are you doing for your bones?
Are you regularly undertaking any activity
that might put a positive stress on them and
maintain or develop bone density? Make a list
of all the activities that would improve
your bone density.*

Your Bones

If you become less active you may find that over time your bones become less resilient and less dense as calcium is lost. The spongy tissue inside the bone can become thinner, and the hard bone on the outside decreases in diameter and thickness. Because of the hormonal changes that take place during menopause, women are more at risk of conditions such as osteoporosis (loss of bone mass), so that they are more susceptible to fractures, shortening of the skeleton and postural problems. Research has been carried out on bone density in active and non-active individuals. It found that the runners' leg bones were stronger than those of the non-runners. It also discovered that the runners' forearms were denser even though no specific work had been undertaken to bring this about. It seems that the whole of the skeleton enjoyed the benefits of exercise.

Studies show that men lose 10 per cent of their bone mass by the time they are 65 and 20 per cent by the age of 80. Women lose 20 per cent by the time they are 60 and 30 per cent by the age of 80. Placing stress on the bones increases bone density and strengthens them. If you suffer from any condition that involves bone loss you need to do weight-bearing exercises. (In some primitive cultures osteoporosis is practically non-existent. This has been attributed to the amount of walking individuals of all ages have to do on a daily basis, which naturally maintains bone density.)

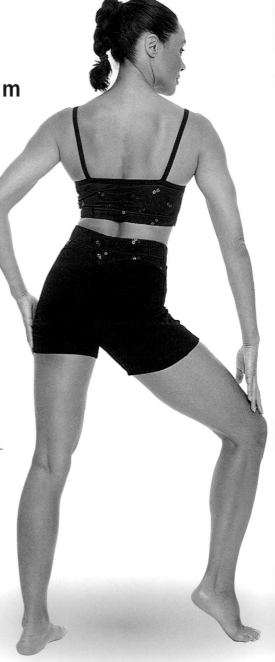

The Central Nervous System

The central nervous system consists of the brain and the spinal cord. One of its functions is to receive messages from our senses and send out the appropriate responses to the body. Changes take place in the nervous system over time. As we become older our responses slow down which can have a similar effect on our movements; balance can also be affected.

The Peripheral Nervous System

The peripheral nervous system is made up of two parts: the somatic system and the autonomic system, which works at an unconscious level to control and regulate involuntary activities such as heart beat, digestion, body temperature, water retention and so on. The autonomic system is also further divided into the sympathetic and parasympathetic systems.

The sympathetic system is responsible for the fight-or-flight response, which acts to increase the work rate of the heart and lungs – in fact it does everything necessary to prepare the body to fight or take flight when it is confronted by a perceived threat or stressful situation. The parasympathetic does the opposite: it slows down the body's physiological processes and promotes a relaxation response in the body.

You'll need a watch or a clock to time yourself doing this balance exercise. Stand with your feet together – you should be barefoot or wearing flat shoes. Close your eyes and place your hands on your hips. Lift your non-dominant foot about six inches off the floor; keep the knee soft. See how long you can hold this position without lowering your foot. Immediately write down the time. Do this exercise every day for a month and see how you much you improve.

The Somatic System

The somatic system operates under your conscious control and consists of sensory fibres, which collect information from the sense organs, and motor fibres, which carry messages to the different parts of the body in order to initiate the responses to our sense impressions.

As we become older we can lose body awareness. If we do not use our motor skills they become less efficient, reaction times slow, balance can be affected and sensory impairments affect our visual, auditory and kinaesthetic systems. However, these processes can be delayed. Being active vastly improves motor skills as well as speed and reaction times. It also promotes the relaxation response, which decreases levels of anxiety and creates a sense of well-being. You can also do exercises to strengthen and fine-tune your senses, so that your vision and hearing improve as you grow older.

Just as you need to exercise the muscles in your body to maintain your strength and suppleness, you also need to keep mentally active to stay young. You can work your mind with the following exercises.

Get yourself into a comfortable position and think of the letter N. Inhale and then touch the back of your front teeth with your tongue. Exhale and make an N sound for about 15 seconds or until you run out of breath. Repeat this three times in the morning, at lunchtime and in the evening before you go to bed.

The exercise above has been tested on people who suffer from mild degrees of deafness. It sharpens the hearing by resonating sound against the eardrum. You can also improve your auditory sense by putting it to good use. Listen to music and to people talking, and spend at least five minutes a day to paying close attention to the sounds around you.

Distance reading. Take some written material and pin it up against the wall. How far away can you stand and still comfortably read it? Mark the place where you are standing. Every day take a step back and over time you will find that you can read it from a greater distance.

Close reading. Take some written material and this time see how close you can hold it and still comfortably read it. As this exercise becomes easier and easier gradually bring it nearer and nearer to you.

20:20 Vision

Over time the lens of the eye becomes less flexible and the muscles around the eyes weaken. The exercises above will improve your range of vision and increase the flexibility and pliability of the lens. (*See* also the Clock exercise in The Yoga Workout on p. 99.)

Your Mental Outlook

You can see how a lack of physical activity has a marked affect on the physical body. We have also established that it is your mental outlook that affects your psychological and biological ages. It has also been discovered that inactivity has an ageing effect on the mind. One of the most prevalent ageing conditions in society today is depression. One in five people suffer from depression, in fact no group runs a higher risk of depression and early death than those individuals who are inactive.

According to researchers, between 42 and 63 per cent of the differences in the specific immune functions of depressed and non-depressed study participants was related to physical activity. Further research explored the link between exercise intensity and depressive symptoms in 663 people. The results showed that the participants tended

Exercise stimulates the release of endorphins which promote a sense of well-being.

663 people. The results showed that the participants tended to be less physically active as they aged. But those who were regularly active reported fewer depressive symptoms; those who became less active were more depresssed.

Depression is a low state of mind that effects people physically, mentally and emotionally. It can be caused biologically by neuro-chemicals that are responsible for mood. It can also be caused by something psychological – a trauma, relationship issues, work problems, financial worries, lack of confidence. The list, unfortunately, is endless.

Depressive symptoms can be general lethargy and lassitude, feelings of helplessness and hopelessness. Depression can afflict us at any time from adolescence onwards but is more common in our later years. Depression and stress-related anxieties have a powerful effect on the way we feel and therefore on the way we look. When we are stressed our bodies adapt by increasing blood pressure, heart and metabolic rates, respiration and blood flow to the muscles. Although this is a natural reaction (it is exactly what happens when fight-or-flight response is activated), when stress is prolonged or triggered frequently it threatens health and well-being and can lead to premature ageing.

Treatment for these conditions often comes in the form of tranquillizers and antidepressants, which restore the chemical balance in the brain. However, when sufferers stop taking tranquillizers or antidepressants, the symptoms can return. This is simply because the cause of the depression or anxiety has not been addressed. Depression and anxiety are often symptoms of something that is going on at a deeper level, and if you do suffer from it I recommended that you talk to someone you can trust – a friend or preferably a professional. It simply helps to uncover hurt, release anxiety and get things off your chest.

But I hope you won't be surprised to learn that your body has its own healing mechanisms to deal with low states of mind and feelings of anxiety and hopelessness. In every doctors' surgery you will find yourself encouraged to be physically active. Exercise stimulates the release of

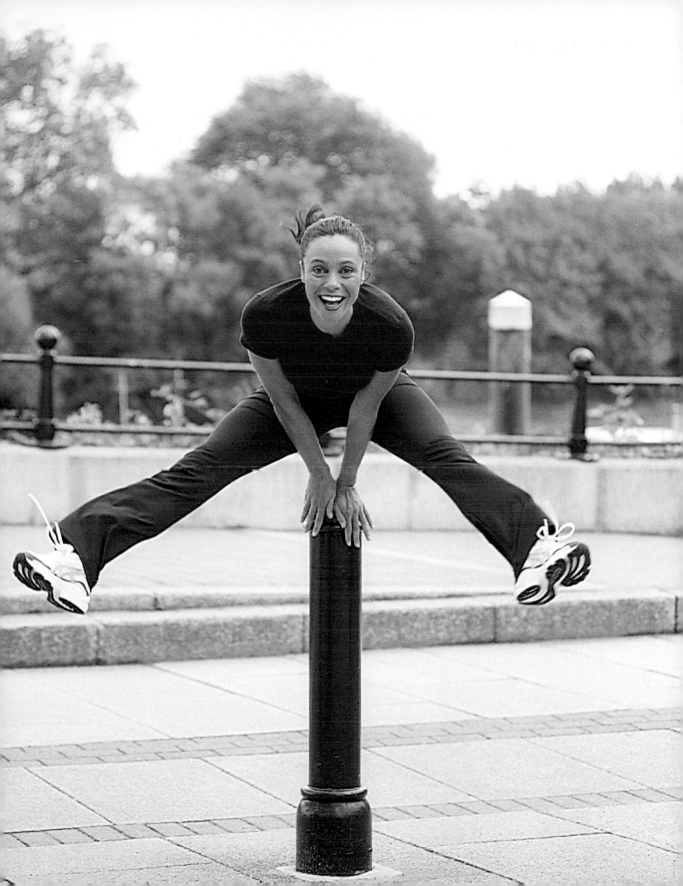

These
'arm aerobics' increase the blood flow
to the brain, which enhances cognitive functioning
and lifts your mood. Sit in a chair or cross-legged on the
floor. Take your arms out to the sides with fingers and palms
tensed into claws. Raise your arms and cross them over your head;
one at a time initially then both together alternating right in
front of left, left in front of right. Bring your arms back to
your sides. Make sure your movements are
smooth and comfortable.

endorphins, which promote a sense of well-being. It also releases negative emotions such as anxiety and anger so that you feel calmer and have more positive energy. Exercise is a great motivator: you develop a sense of achievement and you are lifted out of the feelings of hopelessness and towards setting up goals in life. Exercise also helps you to sleep better and encourages social interaction, which results in greater confidence and self-esteem so that you feel happier about yourself.

Have you lost your natural ability to move your body? Well even if you have it is not too late to relearn it. It is never too late and you can begin to get fit at any age. It will make a huge difference to how you look and feel – most of what we call ageing is avoidable by simply moving our bodies. If you want to look and feel younger then you need to train your body to what it was naturally meant to do.

Sit and relax and take three deep breaths. Repeat the affirmation, 'My body is relaxed', and allow your body to do just that.

Imagine that you are in a cinema facing a giant movie screen. Watch as a picture of you emerges on the screen. Now imagine what you will look like in five years' time if you maintain your current level of activity – and let the image fade away. Now create a picture of you in ten years' time if you maintain your current level of activity – and let the image fade away. And now do the same for 20 years in the future. Notice the changes in your body. Look at the tone and texture of your muscles and your skin. See yourself pinching your skin to measure its elasticity and your body fat level. Feel the firmness of your muscles.

Does this picture provoke a positive feeling? If the answer is 'No' then erase it completely. Replace it with a picture of you as you would like to be – the end-result of exercising consistently for the next 5, 10 or 20 years. Note the tone and texture of your skin and your strong, firm muscles.

How do these new images compare with the originals? Think of three ways to empower yourself to work towards the goal of a younger, stronger, healthier body.

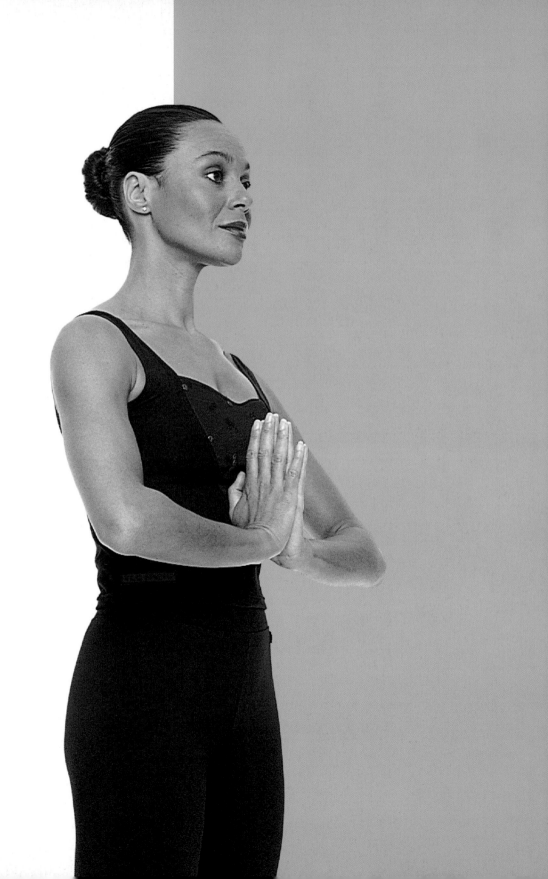

Chapter 5

The Yoga Workout

In stretch and yoga postures it is important to pay attention to your breathing. Aim to breathe evenly, rhythmically and naturally throughout all the postures so that you get a sense of synchronizing the breath and movement together. It is important you breathe in a natural way throughout that suits you. In yoga the tendency is to breathe in and out through the nose. However, again you must do what suits. What is important is that you remember to breathe throughout each range of movements and do not hold your breath.

The Yoga Workout

- Wear comfortable clothing.
- Workout with bare feet.
- Make sure your environment is warm.
- Use a mirror to guide yourself into poses. (When you have learnt the poses work without a mirror).
- Increase body awareness by noticing how you feel and making positive affirmations.
- Postures should not hurt – if there is any strain check your technique.
- Ensure that you practice regularly.
- Work at a pace that is comfortable but challenging.
- Work at a pace that is comfortable but challenging.
- Listen to your body at all times.

Your Breath

Lie on your back in a relaxed and comfortable position. Knees could be bent if you wish. Have a sense of being centred. Breathe in through your nose for four counts and then breathe out for six counts. You may want to take your hand to all your breathing areas the abdomen: the lower ribs and back. Now imagine that your body is a battery that needs recharging. Ensure that you do not enforce the breath. Let it simply come and go. As you breathe in feel the flow of energy filling every cell of your being. As you breathe out have a sense of all impurities leaving your body.

Visualize and Affirm

Now make a positive affirmation to yourself.

- I look forward to my exercises.
- My hamstrings are becoming more and more flexible every day.

Make a commitment to visualize yourself performing each posture correctly.

Full Body Stretch

To stretch the sides of the body

- Lie on your back and bring your hands over your head.
- Inhale as you get into position and exhale as you stretch through to your fingertips.
- Focus on stretching through the right side of your body and press the left heel away, then change sides.
- Feel the stretch along the sides of your body.
- Ensure that you are breathing evenly throughout.

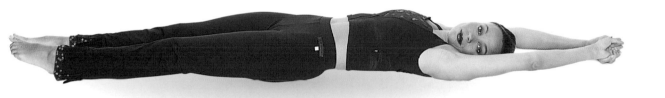

Hug Knees to Chest

To stretch the lower back muscles and back of the neck

- Lying on your back, bend your knees and hug them towards your chest, lifting your head off the ground. You may want to rock your body forward and back.
- Relax the shoulders as you do so. Again breathe naturally throughout.

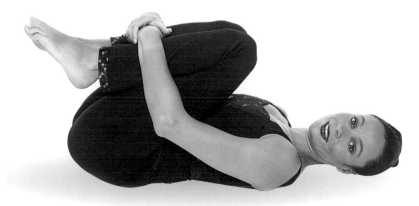

Cat Stretch
To stretch the spine

- Inhale and place your knees under your hips and your hands under your shoulders.
- Exhale and lift up through the spine, stretching like a cat. Make sure your shoulders are relaxed.
- Inhale to release the stretch, then exhale ensuring you maintain a neutral spine.

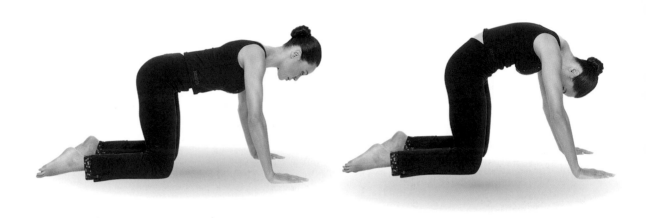

Waist Stretch
To loosen the spine and tighten the abdominal and waist muscles

- Get into the first position above. Inhale and turn to the right bringing your right arm up and out above your head, opening out the chest and shoulders.
- Exhale and feel the twist in the abdomen as you stretch towards the ceiling. Make sure your eye line follows your hand as you stretch.

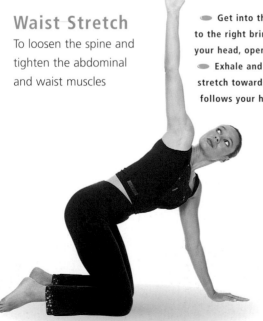

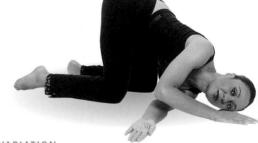

VARIATION

- Slide your right arm underneath the left, travelling with the exhalation as far as you comfortably can. Hold for a few breaths relaxing the shoulders.

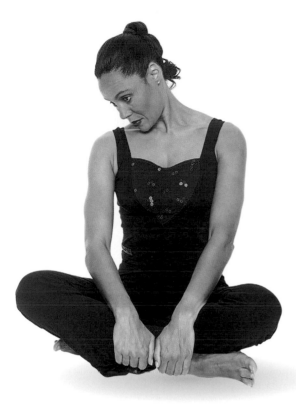

Neck Rolls

To release tension in the neck, shoulders and upper back

- In a sitting position and with your back up against a chair, inhale and look straight ahead of you, then exhale.
- Now drop your chin towards your chest and feel the back of your neck stretching. Hold for a moment and then inhale.
- Gently turn your head to bring your chin to your right shoulder. Exhale and then hold for a moment, looking over your right shoulder.
- Come back to the centre and now turn to the left. Use the same breathing pattern.
- Come back to the centre and inhale. Gently tip your head back (if you have neck problems don't do this one) and exhale. Feel the stretch at the front of the neck.
- Inhale and come back to the centre, then exhale bringing the right ear down towards the right shoulder. Hold for four counts and bring the head to the left shoulder.
- Now repeat this whole sequence as a circling movement. Now change the direction. Inhale and exhale throughout.

The Clock

To strengthen the eye muscles

Your eye muscles can become weak just as any other muscle in the body especially if you spend long periods of time in front of the computer or reading in poor light. The following exercise keeps the eye muscles strong

- Sit in an upright position and spend a moment focusing your attention on your breathing.
- Imagine you are looking at a large clock. See all the numbers on the clock. Now start to pay attention to each number. Allow your eyes to rest on 12 then pause for two counts take them to 1 and so on. Make a full circle. Then do the same anti-clockwise.
- Now gently blink several times to bathe your eyes in their natural fluid.

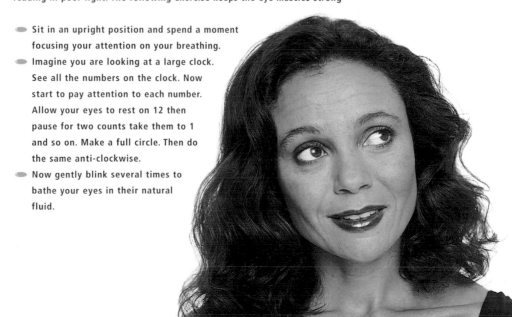

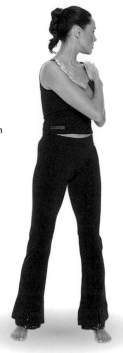

Waist Twist
To warm up the spine

- Stand with you feet hip distance apart, with your hands crossed over your chest.
- Exhale and lift up as you turn to look over your left shoulder and then come back to centre. Repeat five times on each side.

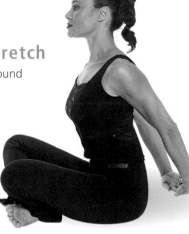

Chest Stretch
To decrease round shoulders

- Sitting on the floor and inhaling take your hands and clasp them behind your back.
- Lean forward exhaling gently and lift up through your chest.
- Looking straight ahead, relax your shoulders and open out your chest. Inhale and now as you exhale and try to lean forward a little more.

Hip Circles
To loosen up the hip joints

- Stand with your feet hip distance apart and your hands on your hips. Keep your knees slightly soft and your spine in a neutral position. Take your hips to the right, forwards, left and back in a circular motion. Repeat five times.
- Now start from the left side and repeat five times.

Shoulder Circles

To loosen the shoulder joints

- Stand with your feet hip distance apart keeping your knees slightly soft. Breathe normally.
- Tighten your abdominal muscles and circle your shoulders up, back and round. Repeat five times.
- Now make bigger circles by leading with your elbows. Repeat five times.

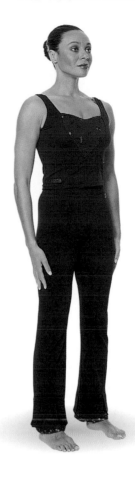

Standing Side Stretch

To stretch the sides of the body

- Stand with your feet hip distance apart keeping your knees slightly soft. Inhale and ensure your hips are facing forward.
- Bring your left arm out to the side and up in line with your body and over. As you exhale feel a sense of lengthening outwards and upwards, thinking taller every time you perform this exercise.
- Repeat five times then change sides.

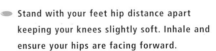

Sun Salutations

Do each of the following exercises slowly and carefully working on quality of movement in each posture. Again ensure you breathe evenly and rhythmically throughout each movement.

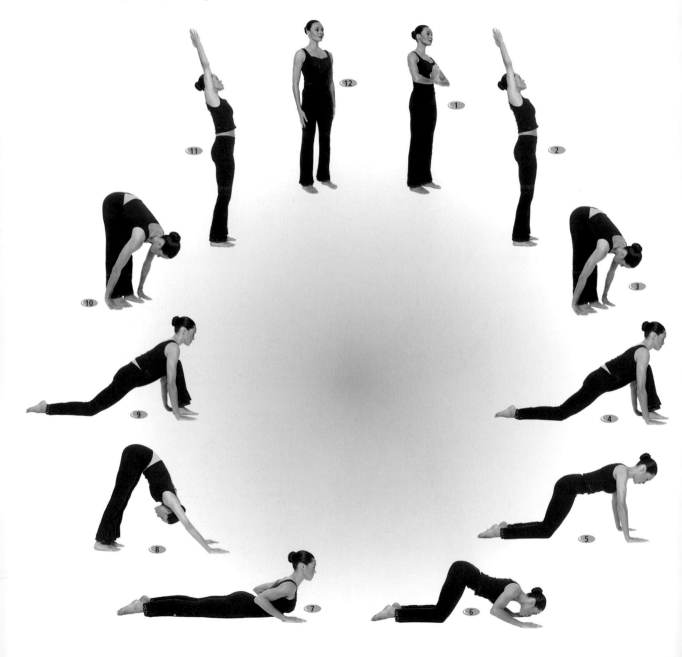

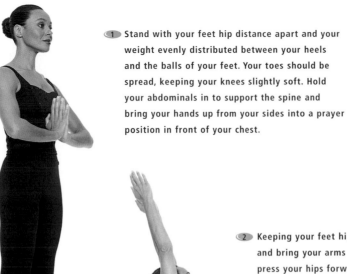

1 Stand with your feet hip distance apart and your weight evenly distributed between your heels and the balls of your feet. Your toes should be spread, keeping your knees slightly soft. Hold your abdominals in to support the spine and bring your hands up from your sides into a prayer position in front of your chest.

2 Keeping your feet hip distance apart, stretch up and bring your arms above your head. Gently press your hips forward leaning your shoulders back. Hold your abdominals in to prevent you from over arching your back. Inhale. Keep your arms alongside your ears and elbows and keep your knees slightly soft. Look straight ahead.

3 As your arms come down from position 2 and with your feet firmly placed on the floor, exhale and bend forward from your hips keeping your knees slightly soft and your head tucked in towards your knees. Bring your hands towards the floor.

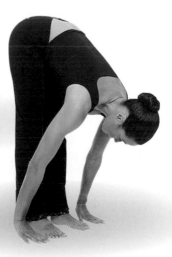

4 Keeping your knees slightly bent stretch the right leg back as far as possible. Dip your right knee to the floor, making sure your hands are next to your feet and your front knee is in line with your ankle. Keep your head in line with your body and look straight ahead. When you are comfortable in this position increase the stretch a little more.

5 Without moving your hands, bring your left leg back and place your left knee next to your right so that both knees are on the floor. Hold your abdominals in and make sure your hands are directly underneath your shoulders.

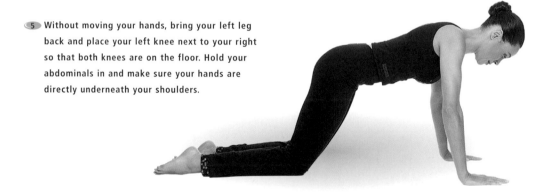

6 Keeping your knees on the ground and your hips still, bring your chest and chin straight down to the floor between your hands. Keep your elbows by your side.

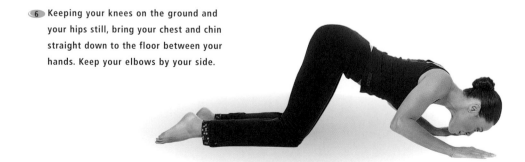

7 Slide your body forwards so that your hips are on the floor but your chest is off the floor. Your hands should be in the same position as before with your elbows slightly bent. Keep your shoulders down and back so there is no tension in the neck. Make sure you don't force, strain or over arch your back. Only come up as far as is comfortable.

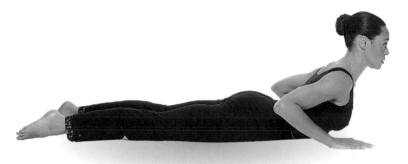

8 Tuck your toes under and without allowing your hands to move from their positions, bring your hips up. Exhale as you push your heels towards the floor. Keep knees slightly soft and drop your head between your arms. Keep your back straight.

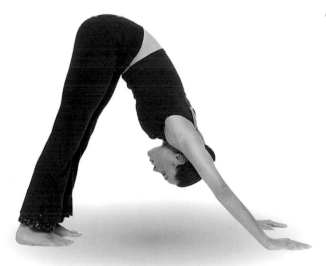

9 Inhale and bring your right foot forward between your hands to return to position 4. Exhale and ensure that your head is in line with your body.

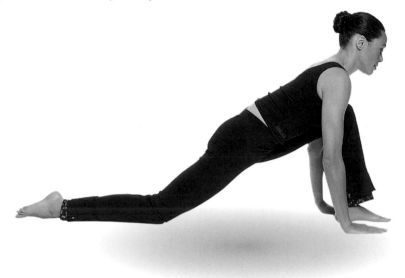

10 Without moving your hands go to position 3. Bring your left foot forwards towards the right foot. Keep your forehead down towards your knees, which are soft. Relax your shoulders and keep the rhythm of your breathing consistent throughout.

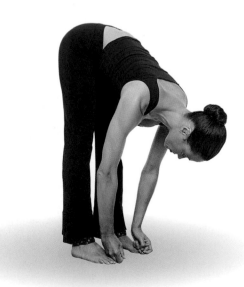

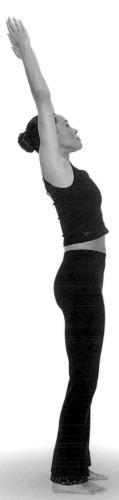

11 Pull your abdominals in and reach your arms forward and lift up through the spine then go back to position 2 stretching your arms up and over your head exhaling with the movement. Now inhale.

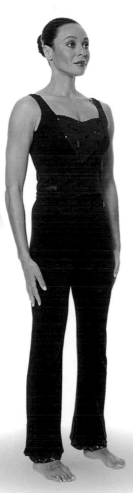

12 Slowly return to an upright relaxed position with your arms resting at the sides of your body. Make sure your weight is evenly distributed and your body is relaxed.

Now repeat the sequence again, leading with the left leg. As you become more familiar with the postures you can increase the speed between transitions.

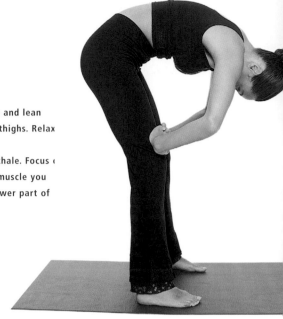

Abdominal Hollowing

To massage the abdominal organs and cleanse the digestive system

- With your feet hip distance apart inhale and lean forward bringing your hands onto your thighs. Relax your abdomen as you inhale.
- Now squeeze in your abdominals and exhale. Focus (tightening the pelvic floor muscle (the muscle you tighten to stop a flow of urine in the lower part of the abdomen).

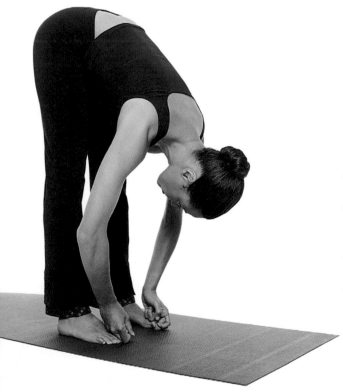

Standing Forward Bend

To loosen the lower back and stretch the back of the legs

- With your feet hip distance apart bend forward from the hips making sure you keep your weight over your feet.
- Bring your chest towards your thighs and your hands down clasping middle and index finger around your big toes. Hold for two breaths.
- Inhale and lift as if to come forward then exhale and go back into position. Hold.
- Repeat five times. Now pull your abdominals in and keep your chest and shoulders open. Bend your knees and again, leading with the hips, come back to the starting position.

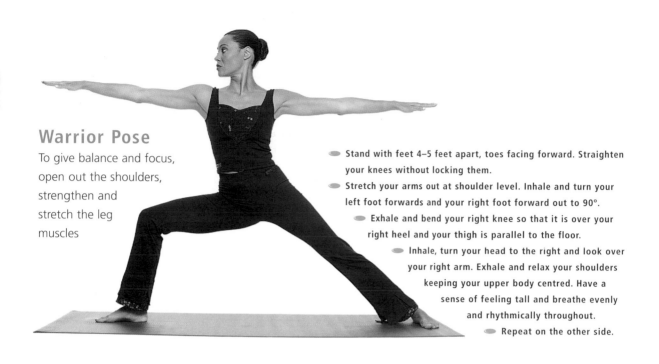

Warrior Pose

To give balance and focus, open out the shoulders, strengthen and stretch the leg muscles

- Stand with feet 4–5 feet apart, toes facing forward. Straighten your knees without locking them.
- Stretch your arms out at shoulder level. Inhale and turn your left foot forwards and your right foot forward out to 90°.
- Exhale and bend your right knee so that it is over your right heel and your thigh is parallel to the floor.
- Inhale, turn your head to the right and look over your right arm. Exhale and relax your shoulders keeping your upper body centred. Have a sense of feeling tall and breathe evenly and rhythmically throughout.
- Repeat on the other side.

Chair Pose

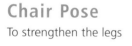

To strengthen the legs

- With your feet hip distance apart face forwards and inhale, stretching your arms over your head with your palms facing each other. Stretch up through the spine keeping your arms in line with your ears. Exhale.
- Press your hips out behind you and bend your knees a third of the way down towards the floor. Sometimes there is a tendency to hold the breath in this pose so make sure you breathe consistently throughout.

The Triangle

To stretch and strengthen the legs and open out the chest and shoulders

- Stand with your feet 3–4 feet apart, toes facing forward. Turn the right foot out 90° and keep the left foot turned in at 15°. Keep your hips facing forward.
- Inhale and stretch your arms out to your sides at shoulder level.
- Exhale and straighten your knees. Without locking them pull up through the thighs and bend sideways towards the right placing the right palm on the lower leg to form a triangle.
- Bring your left arm straight above your left shoulder and reach towards the ceiling. Follow your left hand with your eyeline. Hold.
- Slowly come out and return to the starting position and repeat on the other side.

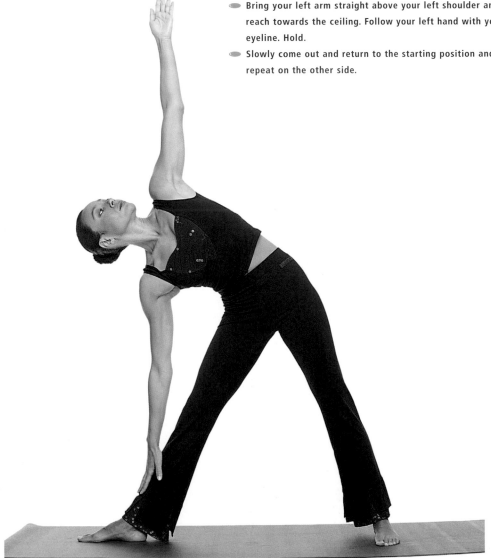

Tree Pose
For balance

You may need to stand up against a wall for support to start with. For balance find a fixed point on which to focus

- Stand with your feet hip distance apart and inhale.
- Shift your weight on to your left leg raise your right foot and rest the heel on the left inner thigh. Exhale.
- Bring your hands together into the prayer pose.
- Inhale and open out the right hip by bringing the right knee out to the side. Exhale. Focus on breathing naturally. Keep your attention on a fixed point to maintain your balance. When you can balance with your hands at your chest with ease bring your arms above your head. Make sure your body remains upright and then hold.

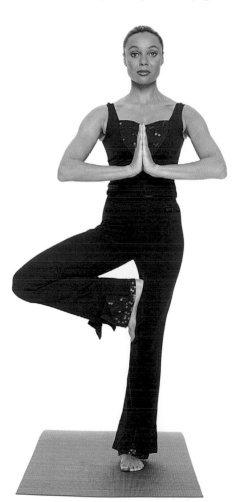
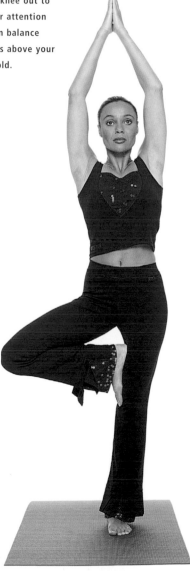

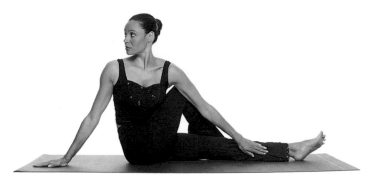

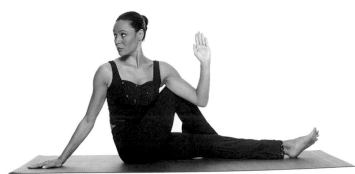

Spinal Twist
To stretch the hamstrings

- Sit with both buttocks on the floor and your legs straight.
- Bend one leg and either place your foot on the floor or by your thigh. Inhale and turn so that your body is in line with your extended leg.
- Exhale and gently ease forward from the hips keeping both buttocks on the floor. Bring the lower abdomen towards your right thigh. Place your hands on the floor for support.

Spinal Twist with Tricep Stretch
To stretch the spine, hips and triceps

- Sit with both buttocks on the floor and your legs straight. Bend and cross your right leg over your left then bend your left knee. Sit up straight keeping your buttocks on the floor.
- Bring your right arm up and bend the elbow so your hand slides down your back.
- Bring your left hand to just below the right elbow to support it.

ADVANCED

- Bring your left hand behind your back to clasp the fingers of the right hand (you might want to use a towel for help).

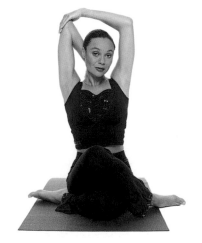

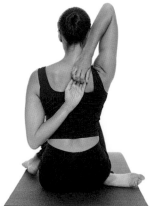

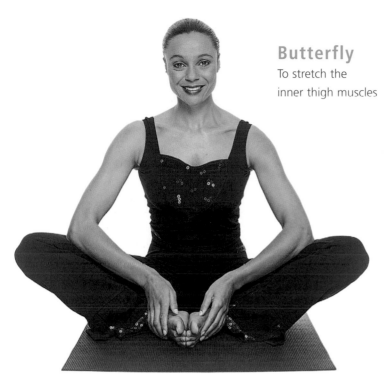

Butterfly

To stretch the
inner thigh muscles

- Sit with the soles of your feet together and both buttocks on the floor. Gently press your knees out to the side and bring your heels towards your groin.
- Open the soles of the feet towards your heart.
- Hold your feet with your hands.
- Lift up through your spine and hold the position.

Single Leg Lift

To strengthen lower back,
buttocks and hamstrings

- Lie in the prone position with your tummy and hips pressed to the floor. Inhale. Place your hands on the floor by your sides and your feet slightly apart. Exhale.
- Gently lift your right leg as far as you comfortably can and hold for 5 counts and then release.
- Inhale and repeat five times then change sides.

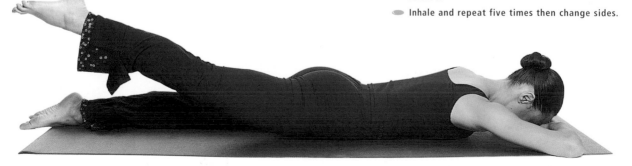

Hip Balancer

To develop the strength
you need to sit up straight

- Sit and bend both knees holding them towards your chest. Lengthen your spine keeping your knees together.
- Raise your feet off the floor to a right angle and bring your hands behind your thighs. If you wish you can then take your hands off your thighs but keep your thighs in line with your body.

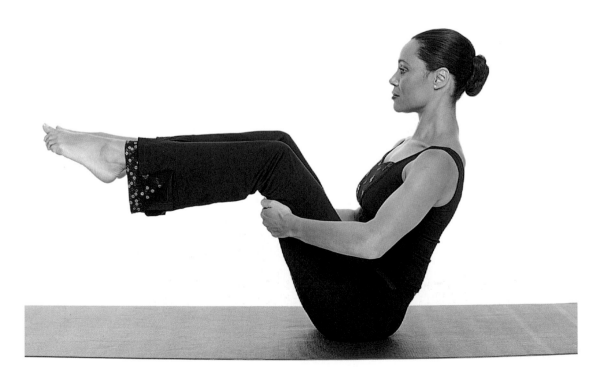

Pigeon Pose

To stretch the front of the thigh and hip flexors

- Kneel on the ground with your right knee bent underneath you and your heel close to your groin. Stretch out your left leg behind you with your knee bent and your foot towards the ceiling.
- Place your left hand down on the floor in front of you and your right hand on your ankle behind you. Keep your head in line with your body, and your body upright. Look straight ahead.

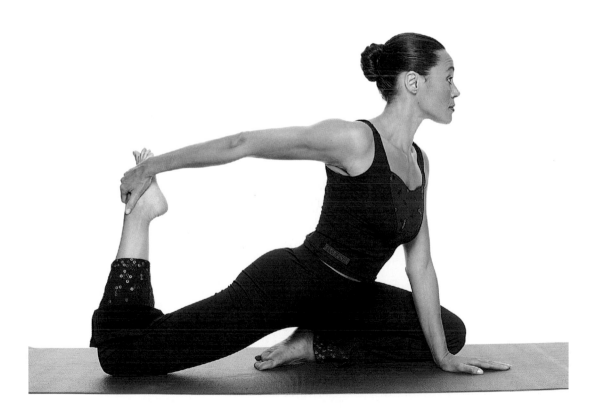

Abdominals

To strengthen the abdominal muscles

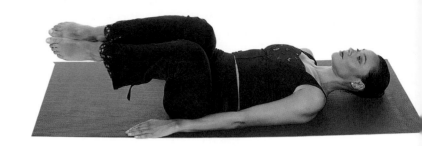

- Lie on your back and bend your knees towards your chest. Inhale and press your naval to your spine. Exhale and gently circle the knees to the left away from the body and then right towards the body. Repeat five times on each side.

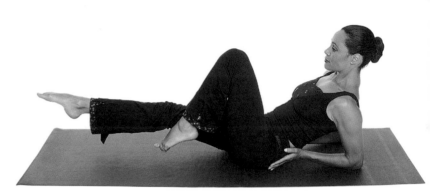

- Lie on your back and go up on to your elbows. (Make sure that they are underneath your shoulders). Extend both legs in front of you.
- Hold your abdominals in and breath evenly and rhythmically making bicycle movements with your legs.

Half Bridge Pose

To strengthen buttocks, back and thighs

- Lie on your back with your knees bent and in line with your toes. Keep your feet flat on the floor, hip width apart. Move your arms down by your sides, with palms on the floor.
- Tilt your pelvis and lift it off the floor towards the ceiling and squeeze your buttock muscles. Keep your shoulders relaxed and interlock your fingers under your buttocks. Keep your knees parallel and press your inner thighs towards each other. Hold for 30 seconds for beginners, 45–60 seconds for advanced.
- Roll down slowly.

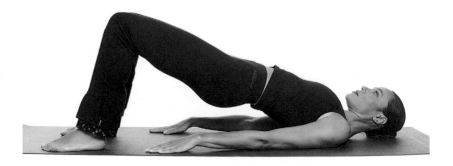

Hip Stretch

To stretch the muscles around the hip and lower back

- Lying on your back with your arms out to your sides and your palms facing down. Keep your right leg straight.
- Bend your left leg placing your left foot on the right inner thigh. Gently turn your left knee towards the right side. Press both your shoulders down and turn your head to the left.

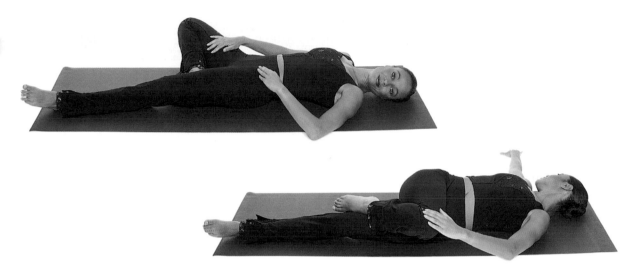

Relaxation

- Go back to a full body stretch, lying on your back in corpse position. Begin focussing your attention on the breath and just allow your mind to follow the rhythm of it. Take your awareness to all the muscles of your body and start to give yourself instruction: I relax my feet. Wait, then visualize the muscles in the feet relaxing. Relax, then affirm my feet are relaxed. Work your way up your body. Make sure the whole of your body relaxes.

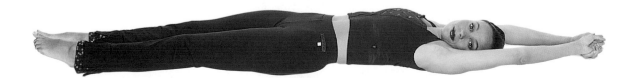

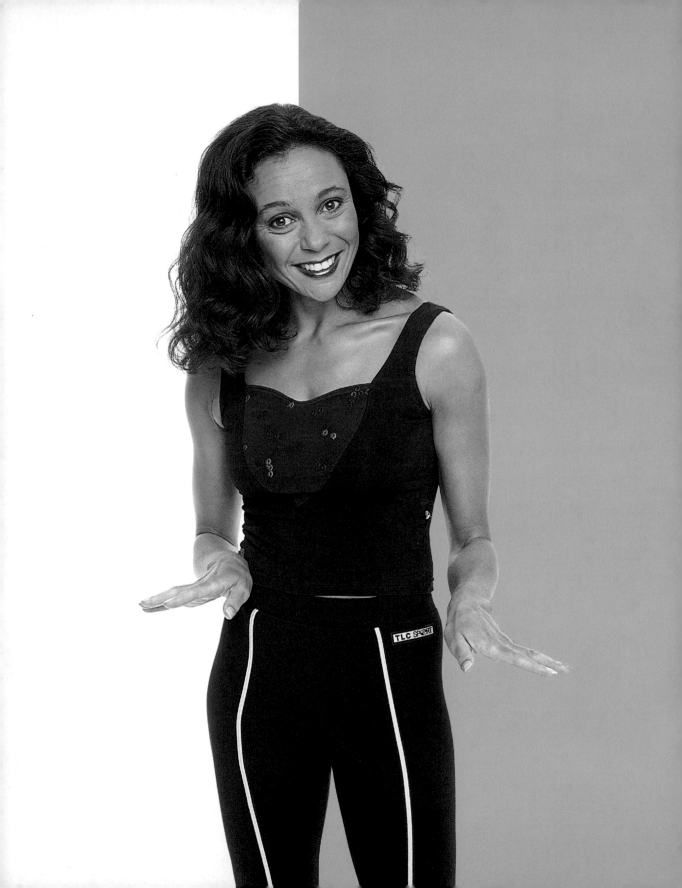

Chapter 6

Stress and Healing

You are now aware of how your mind affects you physically. One of the most common causes of physiological degeneration is stress. Stress is one of the greatest contributors to biological ageing, sapping you of vitality and affecting the way you look and feel. The stress response is an automatic process, an inborn mechanism. When you become stressed your body responds in two ways: it readies itself to fight or take flight. The body adapts by pumping stress hormones into the system so that the heart rate speeds up and blood pressure increases, as does blood flow to the muscles, preparing them for action. Modern life is such that stress can be prolonged and stress hormones continuously pumped into the body.

Stress and Healing

The result of continuous stress is a number of conditions of varying levels of seriousness including heart attacks, diabetes, a weakened immune system, high blood pressure, skin problems and asthma. Ongoing stress can have an effect on your mind and spirit as well. One in four people suffer from mental illnesses like depression and other anxiety disorders.

Essentially it is how you deal with potentially stressful situations that will trigger the stress response – or not. The way you manage your life and the decisions you take will dictate whether yours is a stressful or stress-free lifestyle. For most of us the society that we live in is a 'doing' society. The prevalent belief is that we need constantly to achieve, to succeed in order to survive in a materialistic world. The result of this is often an excess of stress.

It is how you perceive situations that can make them stressful

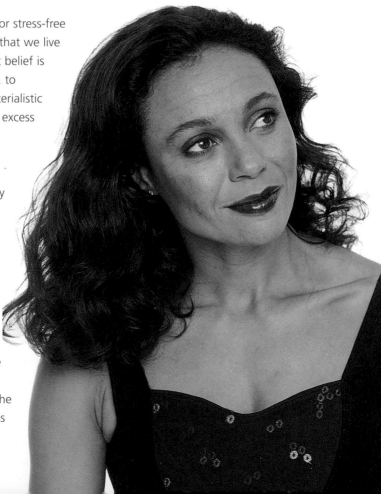

Stress can occur at any age. Teenagers, for example, may be stressed by studying for exams or by the general complexity of life during those years. With time come other commitments such as moving house, building a career, relationships, children, divorce, retirement, bereavement; all – depending on your 'take' on each situation – can trigger the body's stress response. Of course the more you do – the more pressure and responsibility you take on board – the more likely you are to increase stress levels. Minor stresses can be caused by simply driving a car, getting on with people, being on time for work, or worrying about world events reported on television and in newspapers. As was mentioned earlier, living in a transient society means that people now tend to move away from family and friends, so becoming more isolated and focusing on themselves. All of which adds to the pressures on an individual.

Soul Language

Medical research has shown that over 70 per cent of visits to the doctor are due to stress rather than age-related ailments. Doctors are now writing 'lifestyle prescriptions' for regular exercise and better nutrition. Doctors are also encouraging their patients to combat stress spiritually through meditation and prayer. Meditation, progressive relaxation and prayer actually induce the relaxation response, which (as you've probably guessed) is the opposite of the body's stress response. Studies have shown that individuals with a strong faith or who meditate are less likely to suffer from high blood pressure or depression and are likely to have stronger immune systems and live longer. Having faith also improves your ability to cope with illness.

Meditation

As harmful as excessive stress is, your body also has a natural way of getting back into balance: namely the aforementioned relaxation response. You can begin to induce this response by examining the 'doing' part of your life. In other words, do less and be more. We have already addressed this to a certain extent in Chapter 4 by suggesting behaviours that will create lighter, more youthful states of mind. Another route is to explore different methods of relaxation.

Brain Wave Patterns

There are four primary brain wave patterns. The Beta state is the state in which you spend most of your waking time. It is a state of alertness and is associated with critical thought. We frequently switch from the Beta to the Alpha state although we are not always aware of it. When you daydream or contemplate life or drive from A to B without knowing how you've done it, or when you watch a great film or read a good book and are oblivious to what is going on around you – this is your Alpha state. It is a state of serenity and relaxation and detached concentration. You are in the Theta state at least twice a day, usually in the morning just as you are waking or when you are on the brink of your night's sleep. This is the state in which people are often at their most creative, producing ideas and solutions to problems. The Theta state also activates the relaxation response in the body, causing your muscles to relax and your heart rate and breathing to slow down and work at their natural rhythms. The Delta state comes only with deep sleep. In this state we process information through our dreams. It is a period of rejuvenation and cell renewal and is essential for reversing the ageing process.

The most useful states for thinking yourself younger are the Alpha and Theta states. These are associated with practices such as hypnosis, meditation and progressive relaxation. Essentially these three are all the same: states in which body and mind are integrated; they have simply been given different labels. For example, the visualization and suggestion exercises that you performed in self-image chapter are forms of self-hypnosis or light trance. What happens here is that you are directing your mind towards your goal of becoming a younger you. You are actively using the Alpha/Theta states of mind; meditation uses them passively.

Both hypnosis and meditation are ancient practices and are instrumental in allowing the body to heal and rejuvenate physically, mentally and emotionally. 'Hypnosis' may derive from the Greek word for 'sleep', but in fact hypnotized individuals are very much awake and aware of everything going on around them. Meditation derives from the latin word *meditat*, meaning 'to contemplate'. Its purpose is to counteract the mind's tendency to wander and its internal chatter so that you experience things as they really are. When you meditate you are taking your mind to a silent space. At the beginning of this book we saw that everyone has their own map of the world and that the perception of reality - whether it is real, that is to say true, or not – is different for each individual. Meditation allows you to put aside that map and be more in the moment. When you reach your silent space – something that we all badly need to do – body, mind and spirit come together as an integrated whole. Its potential for reversing the effects of ageing are enormous. When you are relaxed and at peace you exude a lighter, more youthful spirit, which results in more youthful behaviour:

- A clearer, more focused mind
- A reversal of the stress response
- A broader perspective
- An aid to rejuvenation and regenerating youthful cells in the body
- A greater connection with others
- A more spiritual experience
- Greater self-awareness
- Enhanced feelings of well-being and enlightenment
- Increased energy and vitality
- A release of emotional blockages
- A sense of freedom within

How to Meditate

Begin by finding a time of day when you know – as far as possible – that you will not be disturbed. Turn off the telephone and put a 'Do Not Disturb' sign on the door. Ensure that you wear comfortable clothing and that you are not hungry or thirsty. Create a space in which you feel at ease and comfortable. You can meditate lying down, sitting down or kneeling. Whichever is most comfortable for you.

You can achieve a true meditative state by focusing either internally or externally. If internally, you can simply pay attention to your breathing and follow it as it comes and goes. You can also focus on a part of the body such as the chest or even contemplate your navel. You may choose to imagine clouds in the sky and follow them in your mind.

You may choose to make your focus external and use candles or an 'altar' or stare at a dim light. You could focus on language and, for example, as you breathe in you repeat a mantra such as 'Peace' and as you breathe out 'Freedom'. Whatever you choose it is essential that you focus your attention and not allow the internal chatter to take over. Allow whatever thoughts enter your head to pass without comment and judgement. Allow your feelings to come and go without suppressing them. Do not will thoughts away, simply allow yourself to be rather than do.

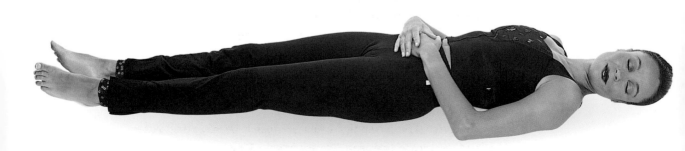

You may find these simple strategies take a little bit of time to get used to. So take the time to adjust to them. Allowing yourself to just be is an essential part of reversing the ageing process and well worth a little time and effort. With a little bit of discipline and regular practice you will notice a new habit forming and you will look forward to achieving this state for longer periods of time. When you practise meditation you will gain a sense of bringing energy into your body. The more you practise the quicker and easier it will be for your to enter a higher level of awareness.

The Energy Field

The Eastern philosophies of which meditation is just one aspect, have long posited the idea that a mysterious force is the basis of our universe. Modern science and theories based on quantum physics now back up the theory that indeed the universe is a vast field of energy. We are not just simply 'static' physical structures, we human beings are part of – surrounded and interpenetrated by – that energy field

Scientists now have the equipment to measure the electrical frequencies of this human energy field. Illness is now slowly being redefined in terms of energy pulses and patterns. Dr William Kilner of St Thomas' Hospital in London designed a special camera that registers the human energy field or 'aura' in 1911. In some Eastern philosophies this energy is called 'prana'; Oriental philosophies call it 'chi'. Western society has also labelled this energy 'life force'. Lynne McTaggart, in her revolutionary book the *The Field*, has explored our existing beliefs about a Newtonian world. We are now discovering a scientific basis for mystical and religious beliefs and proving that there is indeed a field of energy that connects us to each other. McTaggart calls this the 'central engine of our being'.

So how does this theory help us to think ourselves younger? Studies at Yale University have shown that when an organ is healthy it has higher levels of energy and vice versa. The alignment of your energy fields is critical for your health and vitality. Ensuring that your body receives the

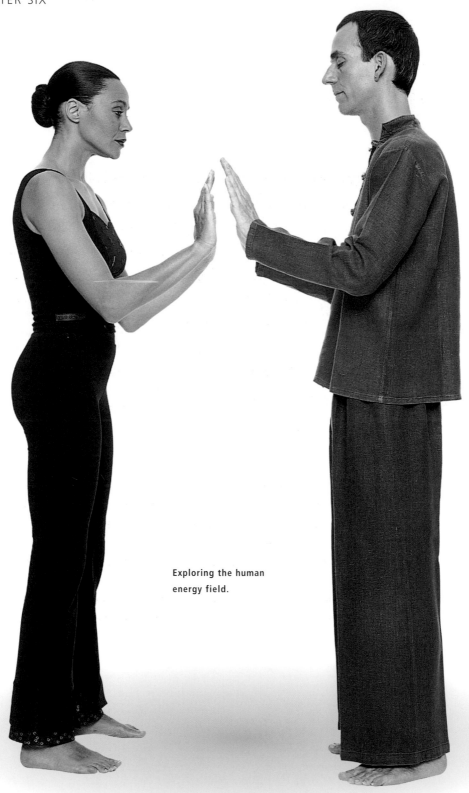

Exploring the human energy field.

You are a human energy field changing all the time.

Find a partner. Stand opposite one another and hold your arms out in front of you, palms facing your partner's. Start just a few inches away from each other and then move a little farther apart. Feel the energy coming off your partner. Now stand to the side of your partner with one hand in front of them and one behind, palms facing in to their body. Begin with your hands at the top of your partner's head and work your way down to their feet. Just be aware of the sensations you experience as you do this. You may find your hands tingling; they may feel warmer or colder. You may experience a pulling or pushing sensation.

right kind of energy – with positive physical, mental and spiritual practises – means that the cells in your body will become younger, healthier and more vibrant. We have already considered some mental and physical exercises that will reverse the ageing process. However, a completely holistic and integrated approach to thinking yourself young should also take your spiritual needs into consideration. We may have got used to thinking of any form of spiritual belief as pretty much obsolete, but in fact spiritual self-awareness has a powerful effect on how the mind and body work.

The Chakras

According to Eastern philosophy we have storehouses for the energy that flows through us. These vibrating energy centres are called chakras, which is derived from the Sanskrit word for 'wheel' or 'circle'. Invisible to the untrained eye, chakras have been described as spinning vortices that regulate body and mind and reflect the state of your health. Situated along the midline of the body, from the coccyx to the crown of your head, there are seven main chakras linked to different parts of the body. Each chakra is also associated with a different psychological state. Some people can see chakras and say that they have different colours. But most people can learn to sense them as they run their hands down the midline of the body; they are indicated by changes in temperature and a tingling in, or increased heaviness or lightness of, your hands.

These chakras transmit life force to every cell in your body. When they are balanced you feel healthy and zestful. Sometimes they become unbalanced, depleted or overcharged, which can result in physical, mental and emotional imbalance. Through meditation and other healing techniques you can channel the flow of energy to maintain your balance. You do this by setting your intention to do so and then directing your energy to the area that needs it.

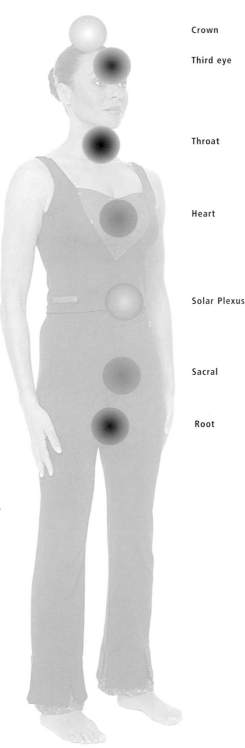

Crown

Third eye

Throat

Heart

Solar Plexus

Sacral

Root

The Seven Major Chakras

ROOT CHAKRA

- Coccyx
- Adrenal glands, kidneys, spinal column
- Groundedness, centredness
- Red

SACRAL CHAKRA

- Reproductive system
- Genitals
- Creativity, sexuality
- Orange

SOLAR PLEXUS CHAKRA

- Navel
- Pancreas, nervous system
- Emotions, will-power
- Yellow

HEART CHAKRA

- Heart
- Thymus
- Compassion, love
- Green

THROAT CHAKRA

- Thyroid
- Communication
- Blue

THIRD EYE CHAKRA

- Between the eyes
- Pituitary gland
- Insight, clarity, imagination
- Purple

CROWN CHAKRA

- Pineal gland
- Higher levels of consciousness
- White

Buddha: 'With our thoughts we make our world.'

Intention

Your thoughts are energy. When you focus your attention on something you are fixing your intention to direct that energy to a given area or target. You drive your energy to meet your intentions. It is now acknowledged that you can use your intention to influence the world even from a distance. At a university in the US studies were carried out into distance healing and prayer. Individuals suffering with acute coronary conditions were made the subject of collective prayer with the intention of healing them. And the patients who were prayed for recovered more quickly than patients who were not. Take this to its logical conclusion and just think how we can influence the world to become ageless through the power of prayer! You don't have to go to church or be even remotely religious to do it. You can have mysticism without organized religion. In fact we may need to address our existing views on religion and unlearn the conditioning that might have prevented us from fully experiencing enlightenment.

Prayer is essentially a meditative state in which you fix your attention on something. When you tap into a higher level of consciousness and form your intentions it is even more powerful because there is no interference from the conscious mind with its limiting beliefs or negative self-talk. Meditation is not always passive, it can be dynamic as well.

So you can set your intention to become more youthful in many ways as you have done already with the exercises in this book. The exercises that follow will further balance your mind and body to reduce stress and put you in touch with the youthful spirit within you.

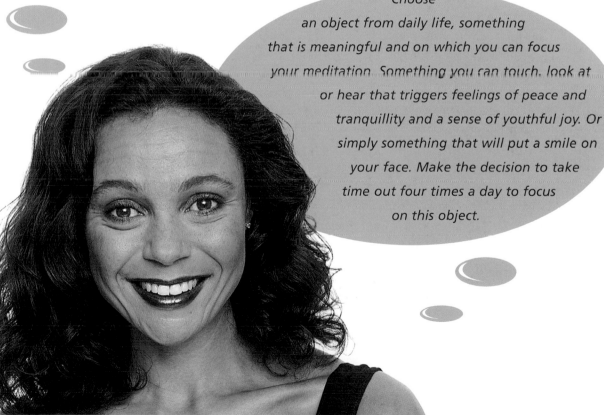

This exercise will bathe you in a shower of light. Sit in a comfortable position in which you can completely relax and spend a few minutes focusing on a mantra or your breathing, or fixing your attention on a candle flame or another object that works as a meditative focus for you. Picture a large bubble above your head filling with liquid light. Now imagine that the bubble bursts and that the light washes through you and the space around you, leaving you feeling cleansed and refreshed. Repeat this five times. Each time retain some of the spilled light, filling your body from the feet up with a vibrant sense of energy.

Choose an object from daily life, something that is meaningful and on which you can focus your meditation. Something you can touch, look at or hear that triggers feelings of peace and tranquillity and a sense of youthful joy. Or simply something that will put a smile on your face. Make the decision to take time out four times a day to focus on this object.

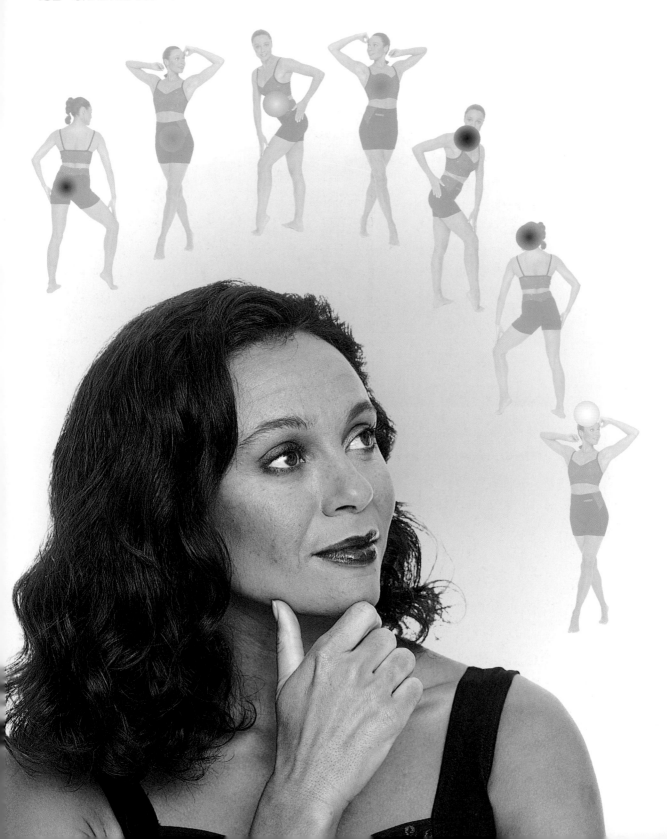

Sit in a comfortable position and take your awareness to all the muscles in your body. Tighten every muscle as you take your awareness to it. Then let it completely relax. When you have fully relaxed your muscles spend a few minutes focusing on your breathing. Let it come and go without trying to control it.

Now focus your attention on all the body's chakras in turn. Start at the root chakra and work your way up to the crown. Sense their presence and get an idea of their condition. See their colours – are they charged and vibrant or are they depleted and sluggish? Set your intention to charge each chakra and make it younger. When you are done, imagine that you are floating out of your body through the red chakra. Spend a moment fixing your intention to send balancing, healing energy into the red chakra.

Now focus on the orange chakra and set your intention to fuel your creative abilities. Move now to the yellow chakra and send healing energy to balance the emotions. Turn to the green chakra and fix your intention to send loving energy into it. Now direct your healing energy to the blue chakra at your throat to improve your communication with yourself and others. Move now to the purple chakra and send clarity and intuition. Lastly take yourself to the white chakra and to the world beyond. Allow yourself to experience a sense of enlightenment, bliss and tranquillity.

When you are ready, travel back down through the chakras and fully experience all their positive energy as you do so. And then return to yourself sitting in the room.

Close your eyes and set your intention to send youthful healing energy to someone who needs it.

Healing

There are many different types of healing. The term can be applied to any practice that addresses the individual as a whole. Many familiar techniques – reflexology, acuppressure, spiritual healing - have the same purpose, which is to make a person feel whole. It is the job of the healer to channel energy from the energy field to the person they are helping.

Healing Hands

The human body has an electromagnetic frequency that is measured in hertz. For the normal human body that frequency is 10_1 Hz. Healers are able to access considerably higher frequencies: up to 10_6 Hz. It has been suggested that master healers such as Sai Baba can conduct energies at least as high as 10_{18} Hz. Almost as high as the frequency of X- or gamma rays!

Hands-on healing is a powerful skill that comes naturally to many who are tuned in to the energy field. It is also a skill that can be learned. Like any art it simply needs a bit of focus and attention. Meditation and deep relaxation will get you to the higher levels of consciouness that significantly increase your ability to channel energy to yourself, your family and your friends. Hands-on healing induces the relaxation response, relaxes muscles so that you look more youthful and sends energy to all the cells of the body. You can also cleanse the body of toxins and release negative emotions and tension. The following is a sequence of hands-on healing positions to balance the chakras.

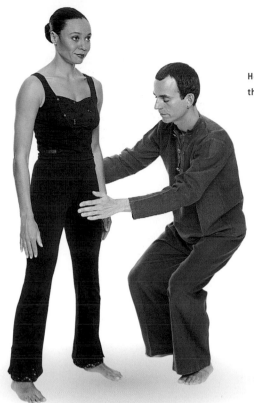

Healing is being sent to the root chakra.

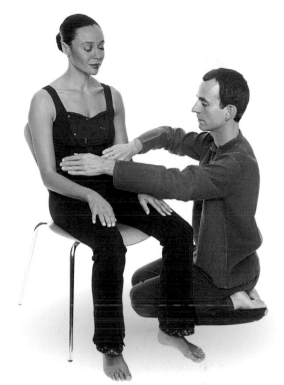

Channelling energy to the solar plexus or the emotional chakra.

Focussing energy on the throat chakra.

Spend a few moments in a meditative state to centre yourself and prepare yourself mentally. Set your intention. Begin by brushing down your energy field from head to foot to soothe and ground yourself. Use the following hand positions as you work through the chakras.

Sit, kneel or lie down. Imagine what form youthful energy might take. Give it a colour, a feeling, a sound. Now direct that youthful energy to the chakras. Move your hands to all the different chakras. Make sure you hold your hands slightly away from your body and press your fingers together to keep the energy focused. Start by spending one minute on each chakra and then increase this over time. Focus on balancing the chakras so that they all work in harmony.

You may find that one chakra needs more attention than the others. If you are particularly stressed, for example, you may want to work on the emotional chakra at the solar plexus. If you have a relationship-related issue you may need to focus on the heart chakra.

Spend a few moments in a meditative state to focus your intention to heal yourself. Begin by breathing into the solar plexus. Now place both hands over your solar plexus and direct healing energy into that area.

An Energetic Facial

You can do this by yourself, but it may be even more relaxing to get a friend to help you. Prepare with a short meditation and fix your intention to radiate youthfulness and vitality from your face.

Sit in front of your partner. Place your hands over their forehead with your thumbs adjoining. Gently move your hands over the face but without touching it, allowing your partner to breathe normally. Now move your hands to different positions on the face and neck, from the forehead to the cheeks and chin.

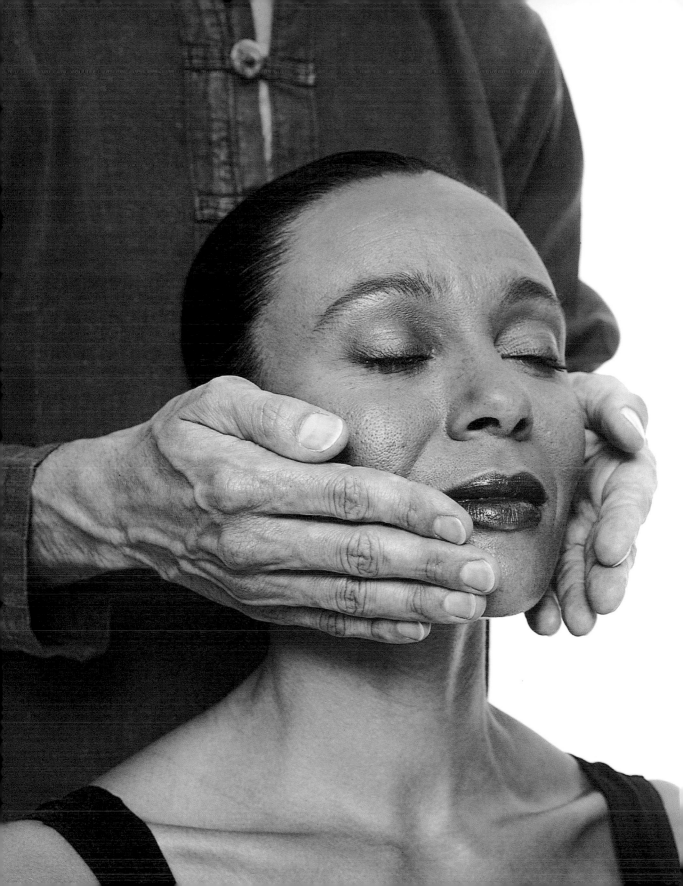

Index

Index

Bibliography

Alex F., MD PhD Dsc Roche, et al, *Human Body Composition*, Human
Kinetics Europe Ltd, 1996

Bandler, Richard *Insider's Guide to Sub-modalities*, Meta Publications,1988

Brennan, Barbara Ann, *Hands of light*, Bantam Books, 1987

Carter, Rita, *Mapping the Mind*, Weidenfeld & Nicolson, 1998

Chopra, Deepak, *Ageless Body, Timeles Mind: A Practical Alternative to
Growing Old*, Rider, 1993

Chopra, Deepak, *Quantum Healing Exploring the Frontiers of Mind, Body
and Spirit*, Bantam, 1989

Dilts, Robert, Hallbom; Tim and Smith, Suzi, *Beliefs: Pathways to Health &
Wellbeing*, Metamorphous Press, 1990

Guinness World Records, Gullane Publishing, 2001

Helmstetter, Shad, *What to Say When You Talk to Yourself*, HarperCollins, 1986

Hodges, Jeffery D, *Sports Mind*, Sports Mind International Institute for Human
Performance Research, 1999

Malina, Robert M. and Bouchard, Malina, *Growth, Maturation, and Physical Activity*,
Human Kinetics Europe Ltd, 1993

McDermott, Ian and O'Connor, Joseph, *NLP and Health*, HarperCollins, 1996

McTaggart, Lynne, *The Field: The Quest for the Secret Force of the Universe*,
HarperCollins, 2001

O'Connor, Joseph, *NLP Workbook*, Thorsons, 2001

Peer, Marisa, *Forever Young: How to Look and Feel Five Years Younger in Ten Days:
A Step By Step Programme*, Michael Joseph, 1997

Pert, Candace, *Molecules of Emotion: Why You Feel the Way You Feel*, Pocket
Books, 1999

Reader's Digest, *Marvels and Mysteries of the Human Mind*, 1992

W, Larry, et al, *ACSM Guidelines for Exercise Testing and Prescription*,. Lippincott
Williams and Wilkins, 1995

YMCA *Exercise for Older People*, 1995

Other Resources

Seear, Michael, The Nine Point Healing Plan

www.med.harvard.edu

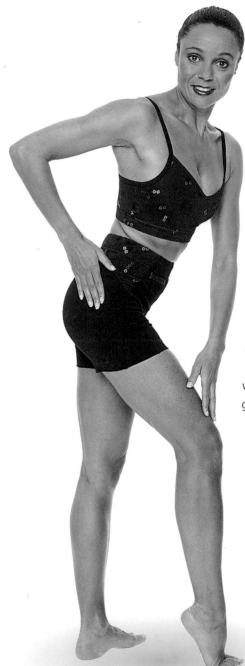

Acknowledgements

The writing of this book has been enjoyable and I would very much like to thank colleagues friends and family for their input. We all have people that we admire and I would very much like to express my appreciation to my own ageing guru Deepak Chopra for his major contribution towards changing the western world view of ageing. I support this vision completely. I recommend his books for a more in-depth reading to the principals of ageing. Thank you to Steve Thomas for his contribution and for the inspiration he has given me to explode the myths around ageism. For his workshops on Ageism in the Workplace go to www.wta.carlson-design.co.uk. Thank you to Reiki Master Michael Kaufmann for assisting in research and for appearing in the healing pictures, reach him on www.nlp-reiki.co.uk. Thanks to yoga teacher Garry Freer at garryfreer@blueyonder.co.uk for overseeing the yoga postures, you can contact him at garryfreer@blueyonder.co.uk. Many thanks to Jane Edmond.

Thank you to Cassell Illustrated for the opportunity to write this book. Especially to Jackie Strachen and Mark Smith for their belief in the concept. Also to Victoria Alers-Hankey for her help. Thanks to Vicky McIvor for being such a fab agent! Thanks to Bill Morton and the photographic team for the photos and also to Martyn Fletcher for the make up. I am also very grateful to the leotard company for providing the stunning outfits that enhance the visual aspect of this book. (The Leotard Company, the thatch, Great Billing Park, Northampton NN3 9BL 01604 416000). Thank you to the fitness work for lending their fitness equipment.